Psychological Care of the Medically Ill:
A Primer in Liaison Psychiatry

Foreword by:
    Morton F. Reiser, M.D.
    Professor and Chairman
    Department of Psychiatry
    Yale University School of Medicine
    New Haven, Connecticut

Introduction by:
    Herbert Weiner, M.D.
    Chairman
    Department of Psychiatry
    Montefiore Hospital and Medical Center

    Professor of Psychiatry and Neuroscience
    Albert Einstein College of Medicine
    Bronx, New York

Epilogue by:
    Martin Cherkasky, M.D.
    President
    Montefiore Hospital and Medical Center

    Associate Dean
    Professor of Community Health
    Albert Einstein College of Medicine
    Bronx, New York

Psychological Care of the Medically Ill:
A Primer in Liaison Psychiatry

James J. Strain, M.D.

Director of Liaison Service
Montefiore Hospital and Medical Center

Associate Clinical Professor of Psychiatry
Albert Einstein College of Medicine
Bronx, New York

Stanley Grossman, M.D.

Associate Attending Psychiatrist
Montefiore Hospital and Medical Center

Assistant Clinical Professor of Psychiatry
Albert Einstein College of Medicine
Bronx, New York

105559

Appleton-Century-Crofts/New York
A Publishing Division of Prentice-Hall, Inc.

Lander College Library
Lander College
Greenwood, S. C. 29646

Library of Congress Cataloging in Publication Data
Main entry under title:

Psychological care of the medically ill.

   1. Medicine, Psychosomatic.   2.   Sick—Psy-
chology.   3.   Medicine and psychology.   I.   Strain,
James J.   II.   Grossman, Stanley.   [DNLM: 1.   Hos-
pitals, Teaching.   2.   Psychophysiologic disorders—
Therapy.   3.   Hospitalization.   WM90 S896p]
RC49.P73   616.08   75-23455
ISBN 0-8385-7947-7

76 77 78 79 / 10 9 8 7 6 5 4 3 2

Printed in the United States of America

Cover design: Morgan Sanders
Adapted from *Man in the Hospital,* a sculpture
by Medardo Rosso. With permission from
the Smithsonian Institution.

Dedicated to our patients, our source of inspiration and continued growth

Contributors

Norman Altman, M.D.

Assistant Professor of Psychiatry,
Bronx Municipal Hospital Center;
Associate Clinical Professor of Psychiatry,
Albert Einstein College of Medicine,
Bronx, New York

Francis D. Baudry, M.D.

Associate Attending Psychiatrist,
Montefiore Hospital and Medical Center;
Associate Clinical Professor of Psychiatry,
Albert Einstein College of Medicine,
Bronx, New York

Jimmie Holland, M.D.

Assistant Director of Liaison Service,
Montefiore Hospital and Medical Center;
Associate Clinical Professor of Psychiatry,
Albert Einstein College of Medicine,
Bronx, New York

Edward J. Sachar, M.D.

Chairman,
Department of Psychiatry,
Professor of Psychiatry and Neuroscience,
Bronx Municipal Hospital Center;
Professor of Psychiatry and Neuroscience,
Albert Einstein College of Medicine,
Bronx, New York

James Spikes, M.D.

Assistant Director of Liaison Service,
Montefiore Hospital and Medical Center;
Associate Clinical Professor of Psychiatry,
Albert Einstein College of Medicine,
Bronx, New York

Alfred Wiener, M.D.

Associate Attending Psychiatrist,
Montefiore Hospital and Medical Center;
Associate Clinical Professor of Psychiatry,
Albert Einstein College of Medicine,
Bronx, New York

Acknowledgments

First and foremost we wish to express our gratitude to Elaine Cohen without whom we feel this book could not have been written. She has been involved in the organization, the writing, and the review of the word by word unfolding of our thesis. Her insight into the problem of translating complicated psychological ideas into cogent statements has been invaluable. Ms. Cohen's familiarity with psychoanalytic concepts and her capacity to help the framers of ideas to develop and then express them has been of great assistance throughout our efforts to create a primer on the psychology of the medically ill.

The Division of Liaison Psychiatry at Montefiore Hospital was established by Morton Reiser and Edward Sachar. From their initial effort the program eventually flourished into a major postgraduate training program in liaison psychiatry. Edward Sachar helped to conceive of a primer that would serve as a handbook and guide for the psychiatric resident in his efforts to provide psychological assistance to the medically and surgically ill. In addition to writing his own chapters, he spent hours in consultation with us as we struggled to find the right target and appropriate level for our primer. We are grateful for his efforts and counsel.

We wish to express our thanks to the liaison fellows who helped to make us aware of the need for such a book. Their ideas mingle with ours; they have been our teachers as well as our students. In a similar vein our ideas are intertwined with other members of the Montefiore liaison faculty: Frank Baudry, Jimmie Holland, Richard Marks, James Spikes, and Alfred Wiener.

It has been our good fortune to have as our hospital, Montefiore, which fosters experimentation toward better patient care. We also acknowledge the support of our own Department of Psychiatry under the leadership of Herbert Weiner, who encouraged us to promote teaching and research of the psychology of the medically ill.

However, for the liaison psychiatrist, the cooperation of his hospital and of his own Department, while valuable, are not sufficient. It was the staff at Montefiore who gave us the opportunity to put our theories into practice. We want to especially thank David Hamerman, Chief of Medicine, his assistant, Sidney Gutstein, and their staff; and the nurses stationed throughout the many hospital services who helped us to implement our goal of better—more holistic—patient care. The Social Service Department, and, in particular, its director, Gerald Beallor and his assistant, Pearl Jordon collaborated with us from the outset in our efforts to foster psychological care for the medical and surgical patient.

We wish to thank our secretaries, Sylvia O'Halloran and Doris Roberts for their devotion and patience throughout the countless drafts of the manuscript; Hilary Evans of Appleton-Century-Crofts, who helped guide our product with forebearance and understanding; and Ruth Kaplan, who assisted in the organization of the reference materials and logs of the liaison clinical experiments.

The experiment on which this book was based was made possible, in part, by a postgraduate liaison fellowship training grant from the National Institute of Mental Health (Psychiatry GP Special Training Grant 5 TO 1 MN13041–04).

James J. Strain
Stanley Grossman

Contents

Contributors, vii
Foreword, xiii
     Morton F. Reiser
Introduction, xv
     Herbert Weiner

PART I
The Conceptual Framework

   Commentary, 1
1 The Precepts of Liaison Psychiatry, 3
2 Psychiatric Assessment in the Medical Setting, 11
3 Psychological Reactions to Medical Illness and Hospitalization, 23
4 Organic Precipitants of Psychological Dysfunction, 37

PART II
Specific Clinical Issues

   Commentary, 51
5 The Current Status of Psychosomatic Medicine, 54
     Edward J. Sachar
6 Evaluating Depression in the Medical Patient, 64
     Edward J. Sachar
7 Hypochondriasis, 76
     Norman Altman
8 The Problem of Pain, 93
     James J. Strain
9 Psychopharmacological Treatment of the Medically Ill, 108
     James J. Strain
10 The Surgical Patient, 123
     Francis D. Baudry and *Alfred Wiener*
11 The Physician's Response to the Dying Patient, 138
     James Spikes and *Jimmie Holland*

PART III
The Evolution of a Liaison Program: A Teaching and Clinical Model

Commentary, 149

12   The Liaison Model of Coronary Heart Disease, 151

13   The Anatomy of the Teaching Hospital, 171
      James J. Strain

14   Building the Alliance, 185
      James J. Strain

Epilogue, 211
      Martin Cherkasky

Index, 215

Foreword

The concepts in this primer reflect the accumulated experience and wisdom of a group of clinicians who had an opportunity to develop at Montefiore Hospital a clinical teaching service in accordance with an idea whose time had come. The idea was to move "psychosomatic medicine" and psychosomatic teaching from its previously sequestered, highly specialized focus on a relatively small group of patients often selected because they suffered from one or more of the "psychosomatic diseases" out into the open field —that is, to develop a program of teaching and training and patient care that would reach into all parts of the hospital. We hoped that such a program would exert some effect on the care of all patients by the teaching hospital staff—of all professions and specialities. Our aim was to persuade the staff to consider the psychological and psychosocial dimensions of illness and hospitalization and help them to realize that the hospital itself is a social system capable of influencing (and being influenced by) the medical course and response to treatment of its patients. The time was right, the place was right, and there were many good professionals already on the staff who had had much experience with traditional consultation psychiatry but were quick to grasp this newer vision of a liaison service.

Broadly speaking, the initial goal of the program was to define and establish an appropriate and effective role of psychiatry in the general hospital and to insure that patients would receive psychologically rational care, which is so essential for optimal medical treatment. What could provide a better setting for the teaching of medical students, house officers (of all specialties), and health care personnel than a hospital so organized? Similarly, what better milieu could one require for the conduct of meaningful clinical and basic research on relationships between mind and body in health and disease?

This is a book about Montefiore. The implementation of the program it describes required not only the best clinical behavioral science and skill, but also a hospital with the soul with which to carry it out. Nevertheless, the philosophy and format the book outlines for the psychological care of medical patients can be adopted by other teaching hospitals. This is an important volume—it deals with the art and the science of medicine and patient care. I am proud to have initiated the program that gave birth to it.

Morton F. Reiser

Introduction

The principles of liaison psychiatry have always been practiced in medicine; it has never been wholly abandoned. For many years, the art of medicine was taught by some remarkable teachers of psychological medicine—Grete Bibring at the Beth Israel Hospital in Boston, the late Stanley Cobb at the Massachusetts General Hospital, and George Engel in Rochester. But one may well ask why liaison psychiatry has flourished lately. Such a question (of recent history) cannot be answered easily—it may take many years to do so. However, one can speculate as to some of the developments that may have operated to bring liaison psychiatry to the fore.

During the 1950's and 1960's the main thrust in medicine was technological, and humanitarianism in medicine was often defined as finding a new antibiotic, antiserum, or vaccine. Although no one can gainsay the great advances that have occurred, each technological innovation was attended by new human problems. For the patient, the intensive care unit was a new and unique environment that evoked psychological stresses that taxed his coping capacities. Similarly, the patient on renal dialysis was exposed to an experience that was not without its physiological and psychological hazards as he repeatedly "walked through the valley of the shadow of death" and delirium.

The great strides that were being made in the technology of medicine gave impetus to social revolution that was occurring at this time. The patient-consumer did not want to be treated by a machine, but by a person. Community groups wanted to participate in medical decisions. And medicine responded to the patient's dissatisfaction with the realization that there was a need to care for his social, personal, and human concerns. The patient wanted persons available to help him adapt to social and political changes in medical practice, to chronic illness and the problems it posed for him and his family. In short, in the medical setting, some of the functions of the priest, minister, or rabbi had to be filled more and more by the physician, nurse, and social worker. And they, in turn, had to be supported by the psychiatrist.

At the same time the psychiatrist, who had been influenced by the writings of Hartmann and Erikson and by medical psychiatrists such as Hamburg, Holmes, Engel, and Rahe, was imbued with the importance of including within his conceptual framework modes of adaptation to change and the conditions that precipitate the onset of illness. Psychiatry and biology had begun to approximate each other; and many biomedical scientists had begun to study problems of brain and behavior. Mutual problems of high interest—cultural, social, ethical, and scientific—had emerged.

The social revolution has also expanded the role of the physician. Thoughtful physicians have become aware of the impact of the environment in inciting illness—whether it be smoking or dietary habits, child-rearing practices or social change. They have developed new insights into the role of personal and social factors in diseases of "unknown etiology."

This book attests to the thought and energy of a group of dedicated physicians under the leadership of James Strain. It also attests to the prescience of two men who epitomize the "new" physician: Martin Cherkasky exemplifies these qualities in his role as the President of a teaching hospital; David Hamerman, Chairman of the Department of Medicine, combines all of the elements of the great physician—the thoughtful and knowledgeable clinician, the scholar, and the research pioneer (in the cellular biology of rheumatoid arthritis). Because of their experience and orientation, they were able to appreciate and encourage the efforts of Dr. Strain and his group to demonstrate that patient care could be improved by the teachings of the liaison psychiatrist and that the care, for instance, of the aged and the chronically ill or dying patient, required some understanding of the social psychology of the patient.

It is to these issues that this book addresses itself. As such, it will contribute to the education of the physician, whatever his stage of development or specialty.

Herbert Weiner

Part I

The Conceptual Framework

Commentary

Liaison psychiatry implies a collaborative medicopsychological approach to the "normal" medically ill patient. However, the means by which this collaborative effort can be fostered have not yet been clearly outlined. Moreover, the psychology of the medically ill patient has not been well formulated.

We believe that the psychoanalytic model of behavior, and, in particular, the formulation of developmental stresses and conflicts, affords an opportunity to develop systematized approaches to the understanding and management of the spectrum of psychological reactions to illness and hospitalization manifested by the "normal" medically ill patient.

Specifically, recent developments in ego psychology enable us to move beyond the stereotyped descriptive models, which explain behavior in such terms as "stages of death and dying," "typical sequences of defensive patterns," and "the uniformity of the reaction of certain character styles to all illnesses." These stereotypes have contributed significantly to the current impasse psychiatrists and internists seem to have reached with respect to their attitudes toward psychological care of the medically ill. In contrast, the concept of the normal stresses of illness and hospitalization and the adaptive and maladaptive reactions they arouse provides the foundation for a dynamic approach that is infinitely more interesting—and more functional—in a hospital setting. In addition, this concept must be supplemented by a knowledge of the psychological correlates of physiological dysfunction, as elucidated by Engel, and the innovative model of preventive intervention, developed by Caplan which extends beyond a focus on the patient to include the patient's caretakers and his milieu. Even the organic brain syndromes, which excite so little interest on the part of both internists and psychiatrists, can be managed more effectively if they are understood within this broad theoretical framework.

Unfortunately, current training programs are not conducive to the assimilation or application of this theoretical framework. All too frequently, the internist has borne the onus for the "mismanagement" of the psychological aspects of medical illness, on the grounds that the core knowledge that would enable him to function effectively in this area is not part of the internist's armamentarium. We feel, however, that this crucial psychological knowledge is not part of the psychiatrist's armamentarium either. The psychiatrist does not know enough about the normal and abnormal psychology of medical illness to offer a meaningful interpretation of the patient's behavior or to formulate appropriate tactics for the management of psychological reactions to medical illness and hospitalization. The need to upgrade residency training programs in medicine, and particularly in psychiatry, to incorporate clinical experience and instruction in this area is a central thesis of this book.

Specifically, our aim in this book is to provide a primer for psychiatric residents—a guide to the understanding and utilization of the theoretical constructs discussed above. Hopefully, this guide will be of value not only to these residents but to all individuals who are involved in the care of patients. The potentially reversible nature of the "acute situational" reactions commonly encountered in the medically ill, and the considerable benefits that accrue from the early detection and treatment of these disturbances before they crystallize into classic, more enduring medicopsychological dysfunctions, such as hypochondriasis or cardiac neurosis—the bane of the doctor's existence—make us hasten to begin our task.

Chapter 1

The Precepts of Liaison Psychiatry

The importance of treating the total patient as a cardinal criterion of medical competence, and the clinical perils of mind–body dualism, are recurrent themes in the professional literature. What has not yet been sufficiently explored is why, given the consensus that seems to exist on this score, this philosophy has not been incorporated and implemented in the hospital setting. Certainly, both the Department of Medicine and the Department of Psychiatry in the contemporary teaching hospital espouse the principle that if treatment is to be effective the patient must be viewed as a "whole" person. But to subscribe to this orientation cannot, in itself, ensure adequate psychological care for medical patients. Humanism must be bolstered by psychological and physiological understanding of normal individual reactions to the stress of illness and hospitalization and by techniques that will facilitate the assimilation and application of this knowledge.

Efforts to develop such techniques will necessarily be based on an awareness of the variables that have precluded adequate psychological care for the medically ill in the past. We believe this deficit can be attributed mainly to four interdependent variables: (1) the revolutions in biology and psychiatry; (2) traditional professional attitudes; (3) current trends in medical and psychiatric training; and (4) systems of patient care in the contemporary teaching hospital. These issues, which are discussed in detail elsewhere in this book, merit brief consideration here, as a preamble to the elucidation of the precepts of liaison psychiatry.

THE REVOLUTIONS IN BIOLOGY AND PSYCHIATRY

The decline of the holistic approach in medicine is, first and foremost, a result of recent advances in biology that have enhanced our understanding of disease mechanisms and enabled the development of new diagnostic and treatment procedures.

This sequence of events, however incongruous it may appear at first glance, is consistent with the history of medicine. There seems to be an inverse relationship between the prominence of the holistic view of man and the availability of medical knowledge: the physicians of ancient Greece, whose knowledge of human physiology was minimal, adopted a truly humanistic approach to their patients. Similarly, St. Bernard, who had little else to offer the "patients" who sought admission to his hospice, relied heavily on the curative properties of reassurance, sympathy, and understanding. The current revolution in biology has caused a predictable swing of the pendulum: the explosion of new knowledge relating to disease mechanisms has resulted in an exclusive preoccupation with the body.

An analogous phenomenon has occurred in psychiatry. Clinical and theoretical advances have characteristically resulted in an increased preoccupation with the mind and a diminution of interest in the body. Gaps in the psychiatrist's knowledge of physiology and of the normal and abnormal psychological reactions to medical illness have compromised his ability to work effectively with medically ill patients.

As is well known, initially Freud's theoretical speculations about the mind called for corresponding extrapolations into the physical sphere. However, a paucity of relevant biological data led to a decision early on to limit his theory of the mind to the psychological parameters of mental life. And the substantial and rapid enrichment of psychoanalytic theory served to reinforce this commitment to the psychological study of man.

This pattern was interrupted briefly in 1943 when Alexander[1] published the results of his pioneer studies of the role of psychological factors (i.e., specific intrapsychic conflicts and specific personality types) in the etiology and the pathogenesis of specific medical illnesses. Had these psychosomatic theories been validated, they might have fostered a more holistic practice of medicine, but subsequent research on Alexander's "specificity" hypotheses proved disappointing.*

Thus, while it is not our intention to minimize the significance of recent major advances in our understanding of the mechanisms and dynamics of human behavior, one is tempted to speculate that these developments may have resulted in an exclusive preoccupation with the mind not only from choice, but also from necessity.

In any event, the argument advanced by several workers that much of

---

* Alexander's hypotheses were based on limited physiological and biochemical knowledge regarding the pathogenesis of the diseases he described. Recent research findings, derived from investigations using different hypotheses, offer more promise for the elucidation of basic psychosomatic mechanisms, but their direct applications to medical practice are not yet apparent.

the mind–body dualism that characterizes current medical and psychiatric practice is a result of an unwillingness and/or inability on the part of both physicians and psychiatrists to "switch" levels of hierarchical explanation seems valid.

TRADITIONAL PROFESSIONAL ATTITUDES

Certain deficits in the internist's traditional professional attitude toward his patients have been reinforced by the revolution in biology. For one, recent advances in this field have led to an increased preoccupation with technical proficiency. Obviously, such proficiency is desirable, but it may also be a barrier to the doctor–patient relationship.

A second, core dimension of the internist's professional attitude toward the patient is his determination not to become emotionally involved, to maintain what Parsons[2] calls an "affective neutrality." This distancing mechanism prevents the medical practitioner from entering into an emotional compact with the patient that might interfere with his objective judgment regarding treatment, and, in doing so is clearly appropriate. Indeed, in certain areas of medical practice, e.g., surgery, it may even be an essential prerequisite of clinical competence, unless, to all intents and purposes, the doctor abandons his patient completely.

As is true of medicine, advances in the behavioral sciences have served to reinforce the psychiatrist's traditional professional attitudes toward his patients: major contributions to the psychiatrist's understanding of the mechanisms and dynamics of behavior have intensified his preoccupation with the diagnosis and treatment of mental and emotional illness. Thus, the tendency to dehumanize the patient by considering just one aspect of his functioning is not limited to the internist. This same tendency is exhibited by those psychiatrists who automatically attribute medical symptoms to psychological factors, who only treat patients by biological methods, or who only treat patients by psychological means.

In addition, the psychiatrist is diverted from the psychological care of medical patients because of the feelings of discomfort characteristically evoked by the prospect of caring for the patient's body—which stems from the deeply ingrained taboo against touching the patient. The maxim that cautions the psychiatrist against personal contact on the grounds that such contact will impede the natural development of the transference is certainly valid when it is applied to the treatment of physically healthy psychiatric patients. However, this attitude must be altered if the psychiatrist is to deal effectively with the medical patient.

THE CURRENT STATUS OF MEDICAL AND PSYCHIATRIC TRAINING

In recent years, a growing number of medical schools have included introductory courses in the behavioral sciences in their curricula, in the expectation that such courses will facilitate the student's understanding of his patient's psychological needs. However, theoretical knowledge of the origins and manifestations of psychological disturbances cannot, in itself, assure adequate psychological care of the individual patient. The student will achieve competence in this area only if he is given an opportunity to apply these theoretical constructs in a clinical setting. Unfortunately, the educational process begun in medical school is not continued in the teaching hospital. During the crucial period of his medical apprenticeship, when the new doctor is in the process of developing the professional orientation that will determine the form and quality of his future medical practice, he is exposed to situations in which the patient's physiological functioning has primacy over all other considerations.

The "good" medical patient, for teaching purposes, is one who suffers from a discrete, reversible medical dysfunction, which, ideally, is also complex, unique, and dramatic. Typically, the resident's mentors attach major importance to his ability to diagnose and treat such patients successfully. Conversely, his teachers place minimum value on the resident's ability to deal effectively with the "bread and butter" physical and psychological problems he will encounter once he has completed his training, despite the frequency with which these occur. Psychological reactions to a myocardial infarction, the constant complaining reactions to illness and body dysfunction, the general, and often irreversible, deterioration of the elderly rank low on the list of teaching priorities.

Similar and parallel deficits exist in psychiatric training. The psychiatric resident's knowledge of behavior is supplemented by the basic knowledge of physiology he acquired in medical school. But his medical knowledge is of little value if he is not given an opportunity to apply it in a clinical setting. Eliminating the internship means that the only contact the psychiatric resident may have with physical issues is his initial work-up of the psychiatric inpatient.*

Reliance on the "good" psychiatric patient for teaching purposes serves to further deflect the resident's attention from the medically ill. The "good" patient in psychiatry is the patient with a discrete neurotic disorder, who has sufficient ego strength to explore his unconscious psychological conflicts and fantasies. The resident's knowledge of the mechanisms and dynamics

---

* Educators have become increasingly aware of the disadvantages of this training format, and recommendations for its revision are currently under consideration.

of behavior is based primarily on his experience with patients who require long-term psychotherapy and, to a lesser degree, on his experience with patients who have been hospitalized for an acute, clearly defined psychiatric disability. These are the cases his teachers and supervisors want to hear about.

These factors intensify the psychiatrist's reluctance to care for the patient whose physical symptoms are caused, or complicated, by emotional factors; who suffers from chronic pain that may be psychogenic in part; for the hypochondriacal patient; and for the dying patient.

SYSTEMS OF PATIENT CARE IN THE CONTEMPORARY TEACHING HOSPITAL

Bureaucratized systems of patient care limit the internist's opportunities to relate to the patient as a human being and to gain an awareness and understanding of his psychological responses to the stress of medical illness.

The frequency with which the hospital staff rotates precludes their prolonged contact with patients. Patients are rotated as well. They may be moved from one hospital setting to another to ensure their optimal technical care. Furthermore, there is a growing trend toward shorter hospital stays. Internists and ancillary personnel, who recognize that their contact will be transitory, are not strongly motivated to form meaningful relationships with the patient, or even with each other. Furthermore, their heavy workloads and the pressure placed on them to function with maximum efficiency limit their opportunity to promote such relationships.

The psychiatrist has even less opportunity to relate to patients on the medical service. Typically, he visits the medical ward only when a consultation is requested.

Thus, in their present form, systems of patient care reflect the philosophy that governs training in medicine and psychiatry. In addition, they operate to implement administrative policies that help to ensure the hospital's economic survival. Unfortunately, however, they also contribute to the devaluation of the doctor–patient relationship, which is the crux of "good" medical practice.

These four variables—recent major advances in medicine and psychiatry, traditional professional attitudes, the content and orientation of medical and psychiatric training programs, and current systems of patient care— explain in part the failure to implement a holistic approach which is accepted as the sine qua non of clinical competence. Above all, consideration of these variables permits certain recommendations as to the task of the liaison psychiatrist.

THE FUNCTION OF THE LIAISON PSYCHIATRIST

Actually, the fact that psychological reactions to medical illness are poorly understood and, by and large, undertreated, has long been recognized. Physicians in a variety of specialties have established innovative approaches to this problem. Cope[3] has written extensively on the psychological needs of the surgical patient; Ham[4] helped to establish a radically new medical training program at Western Reserve, designed to foster holistic ideals. Psychiatrists, such as Engel,[5] Romano,[6] and Bibring and Kahana[7] have made notable efforts to provide medical students and residents with the core knowledge of behavior that would enhance their awareness of the "humanness" of their patients. Levine[8] has emphasized the importance of a program that would train psychiatrists, as well as internists, to view and understand the patient as an integral unit.

In formulating our concept of the role of the liaison psychiatrist, we have drawn heavily on the pioneer contributions of these workers. In the final analysis, however, the solution we have proposed to the problem of inadequate psychological care of the medically ill is the product of our own experience in this area. We have concluded, on the basis of this experience, that it is unrealistic to assume that any teaching program can guarantee that all physicians will be competent to provide adequate psychological care for all their patients. Technical proficiency in surgery, for example, may, as noted earlier, depend on the surgeon's ability to isolate himself from the patient as a person. With respect to individual considerations, Balint[9] found that many highly motivated internists who attended psychological seminars over a period of two to three years showed only a limited capacity at the end of this period to understand psychological issues and to provide supportive psychotherapy.*

In light of these considerations, the implementation of a team approach to psychological care of the medical patient may be a more realistic goal than the construction of a program designed to enable the internist to function autonomously in this area. Such an approach would utilize the knowledge and skills of the psychiatrist, who would join with the internist, the nurse, and social service personnel, to provide psychological care for the

---

* It should be noted, however, that the criteria on which Balint based this conclusion were more applicable to psychiatric residents than to internists. Perhaps he was trying to train psychotherapists, rather than implement his stated goals: to provide internists with the knowledge and skills that would enable them to recognize depression, organic mental syndromes, anxiety, and somatic equivalents; to manage the difficult, uncooperative, hypochondriacal patient; and to help the medical patient to cope with the psychological suffering that accompanies illness, loss, abandonment, and pain.

medical patient. The degree to which each member of the team participated in this effort would depend on the worker's specialty and his individual ability and aptitude. Depending on their ability to do so, some internists would eventually be able to function independently in this area. And, in that event, the psychiatrist's active participation as a member of the team might become unnecessary, although he would continue to be available as a resource person. At the least, the team is a step toward ensuring a most favorable environment for the maintenance and restoration of the psychological well-being of the hospitalized population.

As the "prime mover" of the team approach to the psychological care of the medical patient, the psychiatrist must develop the following capacities:

1. He must be taught how to conduct a proper consultation, which means that his training must be expanded to include more extensive instruction in the psychological reactions of the medically ill.
2. He must develop techniques that will enable him to transmit his knowledge and skills to his medical colleagues.
3. Finally, in our schema, the psychiatrist must learn to deal effectively with the staff and administration in order to enlist their support of his efforts to produce structural changes in patient care and nursing so that the hospital milieu will reflect a responsiveness to the psychological needs of the medically ill.

Within this conceptual framework, the goals of liaison psychiatry can be defined with greater specificity. In contrast to the routine consultation method, liaison psychiatry seeks to enhance the quality of psychological care for the medically ill by using Caplan's model of prevention,[10] that is, by anticipating and preventing the development of psychological symptoms (primary prevention); by treating such symptoms after they have developed (secondary prevention); and by rehabilitating patients who have manifested such symptoms, in order to prevent their recurrence (tertiary prevention). In addition, the liaison psychiatrist differs from the psychiatric consultant in that the liaison psychiatrist participates in case detection rather than awaiting referral, clarifies the status of the caretaker and the patient (using the chart, doctor, nurse, family, and patient as data sources), and provides an ongoing educational program that promotes more autonomous functioning by medical, surgical, and nursing personnel with regard to handling their patient's psychological needs.

Essentially, the liaison psychiatrist achieves these aims by developing a core knowledge of the psychological aspects of medical illness and by building alliances that will enable him to effectively transmit this knowledge to the patient's caretakers.

REFERENCES

1. Alexander F: Fundamental concepts of psychosomatic research: psychogenesis, conversion, specificity. Psychosom Med 5:205, 1943
2. Parsons T: The Social System. Glencoe, Free Press of Glencoe, 1951, pp. 428–473
3. Cope O, Zacharias J: Medical education reconsidered. Endicott House Summer Study on Medical Education. Philadelphia, Lippincott, 1966.
4. Ham TH: Personal communication
5. Engel G: Psychological Development in Health and Disease. Philadelphia, Saunders, 1962
6. Romano J: Teaching of psychiatry to medical students. Lancet 2:93, 1961
7. Bibring G, Kahana R: Lectures in Medical Psychology. New York, International Universities Press, 1968
8. Ross, WD, Levine, M: Training in psychosomatic medicine. In F. Deutsch (ed): Advances in Psychosomatic Medicine, Vol 4. New York, Hafner, 1964, pp. 14–22
9. Balint M: The Doctor, Patient and His Illness. New York, International Universities Press, 1957
10. Caplan G: Principles of Preventive Psychiatry. New York, Basic Books, 1961

BIBLIOGRAPHY

Kimball CP: Role of liaison psychiatrist in teaching medical students. Comp Psych 12:5, 1971.

Lipowski ZJ: Review of consultation psychiatry and psychosomatic medicine. I. General principles. Psychosom Med 29(2):153–171, 1967.

Lipowski ZJ: Review of consultation psychiatry and psychosomatic medicine. II. Clinical aspects. Psychosom Med 29(3):201–224, 1967.

Lipowski ZJ: Review of consultation psychiatry and psychosomatic medicine. III. Theoretical issues. Psychosom Med 30(4):395–422, 1968.

Chapter 2

Psychiatric Assessment in the Medical Setting

Regardless of the treatment setting, the psychiatrist's initial efforts will necessarily center on the accumulation of data that will enable him to accurately assess the nature, severity, and possible psychological and/or organic determinants of the patient's presenting problem. However, important distinctions can be made between psychiatric assessment in the medical setting and psychiatric evaluation in the traditional setting. These distinctions are dictated by the different characteristics—and needs—of the patient populations seen in these settings. In the traditional treatment setting the psychiatrist deals with patients whose presenting complaints are indicative of the presence of psychopathology of varying severity; who know they are psychologically ill (although they may ascribe their symptoms to physical factors); and who, for the most part, seek psychiatric help on their own initiative. In contrast, normal medically ill patients may not have a typical psychiatric presenting complaint. In fact, they may not be consciously aware of the fears, anger, anxiety, and other reactions that their illness and/or hospitalization have evoked, and they are just as likely to be oblivious to the fact that their consequent behavior has taxed the patience of the hospital staff and, in some instances, has led to growing antagonism on the part of the staff. Nor are they apt to seek psychiatric help on their own initiative.

Consequently, psychiatric assessment of the hospitalized patient is unique with respect to certain general aspects of this procedure (i.e., the content of the patient interview, the issue of confidentiality, the setting in which the interview is conducted, the mode of referral), and with respect to the scope of the interview in particular.

GENERAL ISSUES

To begin with, the interview of the nonpsychiatric patient focuses on the immediate determinants of his presenting problem: his medical diagnosis and prognosis, the psychological climate of the hospital, his relationship with his internist and the hospital staff, and the psychological stresses these elicit. Second, with regard to the issue of confidentiality, since the psychiatrist relies on the patient's caretakers to implement his therapeutic recommendations, he must share with them certain of his findings, and must so inform the patient. As to the third issue, the setting in which the interview is conducted, the medical ward does not offer the tranquility, privacy, and comfort that are associated with the traditional treatment setting. The appearance of the patient, the fact that he may be in pain, the noise, the medical apparatus—all distract both the psychiatrist and the patient from the business at hand. Furthermore, the fact that the patient is not self-referred and may not be motivated may prove to be still another obstacle to the psychiatrist's efforts to assess his problem.

THE SCOPE OF THE INTERVIEW

The psychiatrist proceeds on the premise that his patient's psychological symptoms can be fully understood only if they are considered in relation to the nature and severity of his medical illness and to the hospital environment. It is this complex interrelationship between psychological and physiological variables that sets the tone for evaluation and treatment of the medical patient.

At the same time, the techniques used in the medical setting to accumulate data that will enable an accurate assessment of the patient's psychological problem and its determinants are not limited to the classic model of the interview, conducted within the framework of the doctor–patient dyad. The psychiatrist bases his final assessment of the patient's psychological functioning and his treatment recommendations on data derived directly from the following sources: (1) the request for psychiatric consultation, (2) the doctor, (3) the patient's chart, (4) the nurse, (5) the patient's family, (6) the ward culture, (7) and, finally, the patient himself.

When the consultation is conducted systematically, the psychiatrist is able to assimilate a great deal of information about the patient before he actually interviews him. His mental image of the patient, from both a psychological and a physiological point of view, and of the patient's caretakers expands at every stage of the assessment. However, the psychiatrist must remain flexible in his approach. For example, if he is able to determine the nature and precipitants of the patient's problem and come to some decision regarding management on the basis of information provided solely by the internist, it may not be necessary for him to interview the patient. Similarly, if the internist or the nurse is in contact with the patient's family and is able to provide the psychiatrist with the information he would normally elicit directly, he may not have to actually see the family himself. The "formula" for the expanded psychiatric interview as outlined below is presented for its practical value.

MODEL OF THE EXPANDED PSYCHIATRIC INTERVIEW

Evaluating the Request for Psychiatric Consultation

Psychiatric assessment begins with an evaluation of the request for consultation. Routine data may actually convey important information about the patient's psychological problem. The psychiatrist learns from the request whether the patient is a surgical or medical patient, whether he is in an intensive care unit or on a general ward, and how long he has been in the hospital.

The wording of the request, which also seems banal on the surface, may provide important first clues to the doctor's attitude toward his patient. Focused, concisely stated requests for psychiatric consultation frequently indicate that the doctor has, in fact, already decided what should be done. One request that read: "Patient is depressed, suicidal, and needs to be transferred," accurately reflected closure on the part of the doctor and a desire to transfer responsibility for the patient. In contrast, another request that read: "Please evaluate patient for bizarre behavior," reflected the doctor's uncertainty and desire for help. Mendelson and Meyer[1] found that less well-focused requests with more vaguely stated reasons for referral usually came from doctors who were more confused and therefore more receptive to the psychiatrist's suggestions.

Evaluating the Doctor

In general, the psychiatrist adheres to certain cardinal principles in his relationship with the internist: He tries to find the best way to help the internist to use his capacity for empathy and his inherent dedication to the patient, and to convince him of the value of what he can do to foster the patient's psychological well-being. On the other hand, the psychiatrist recognizes that he must respect and work with the internist's limitations.

At times, these "limitations" must be identified with greater specificity.

It may be necessary, for example, to further assess the internist's ability to think in psychological terms and to empathize with the emotional needs of the patient. At other times, it is important to establish whether a particular patient is making the internist anxious, and if so, why.

The psychiatrist cannot afford to endow the internist with insights he doesn't possess and expect him to manage psychological situations that are currently beyond him.

> When the psychiatrist saw the doctor who had initiated a request for consultation for a depressed patient, it immediately became apparent that it was the doctor who was despondent. Although Dr. N. realized they would prolong the patient's life, she was afraid to administer "poisons" (immunosuppressant drugs) to her young, healthy-looking patient, who, in fact, was dying from leukemia. Dr. N. had expressed her anxiety and depression through the medium of the consultation request.

Dr. N. had not been consciously aware of how upset she was, or of the source of her anxiety and despondency, before she discussed the situation with the psychiatrist. However, she was aware of the fact that her consequent inability to talk with the patient had increased his concern and anxiety. After she had expressed her feelings about her patient, she recognized that she could not continue to function as his doctor. Dr. N. was clearly overwhelmed by her patient.

However, a tendency to automatically discount the internist's capacity to deal with his patient's psychological needs may prove equally unfortunate.

> Mr. M., an Englishman in his 50s, suffered from chronic leukemia that was fairly asymptomatic, except for one acute episode, marked by weakness, which had required his hospitalization. The patient, who had spent most of his life at sea, had little capacity to relate to others—even his wife—on an intimate level. He had defended against closeness and passive longings by cultivating the image of a bon vivant, and even after the onset of his illness continued to maintain that façade. His underlying melancholy, associated with his fears of weakness and death, became manifest during the brief exacerbation of his illness.
>
> Mr. M.'s physician, a sensitive oncologist, dealt with him on a man-to-man basis and made no attempt to make him aware of his feelings. However, the psychiatrist who had seen him while he was despondent during his hospitalization recommended that the internist probe the patient's defenses. The psychiatrist based the recommendation on his belief that Mr. M. had an underlying depression that should be explored. Although the physician was reluctant to do so, such an attempt was made—and produced only

increased defensiveness in the patient, a reinforcement of his image, and some agitation.

In making his recommendations, the psychiatrist had been following the "modern" therapeutic formula, which fails to take into account the individual's psychological makeup. On the other hand, the internist had a "feel" for his patient. Once this became apparent, the psychiatrist and the internist agreed that the defenses the patient had erected against his responses to his illness should be respected and strengthened until they could no longer withstand the reality of his physical symptoms.

In a third case the psychiatrist was able to accurately evaluate the seemingly paradoxical ability of a young, inexperienced intern to fulfill the psychological needs of a patient who was a senior attending at the hospital.

> Dr. S. had a fever of undetermined origin and a probable occult neoplasm. While awaiting the results of diagnostic tests, the patient became increasingly anxious. His private physician, who was a close friend, was understandably distressed about his condition, to the extent that he could not discuss the situation with Dr. S., or, in fact, talk with him at all.
>
> When Dr. S. was subsequently presented at medical rounds, he expressed his fear and his intense desire to talk to someone. The psychiatrist felt that Dr. S. would form an immediate relationship with anyone who would listen. Consequently, when a young intern expressed an interest in Dr. S., and wondered whether he could help an older patient, and a physician at that, the psychiatrist encouraged him to try. The patient's psychological status improved significantly as a result.

It is the exquisite tailoring of the consultation not only to the needs of the patient, but also to the needs and capacities of the doctor, that is the hallmark of liaison methodology.

Evaluating the Chart

The chart, like the request for consultation, contains both explicit and implicit psychological and physiological data. The psychiatrist takes a "bird's-eye view" of the chart, correlating changes in the patient's mood and behavior with changes in his chemistries, specific medications, diagnosis, treatment procedures, with changes in ward personnel, and with visits from specific family members and friends.

When the doctor's observations of a patient's behavior are at odds with the observations of the nurses, the chart may highlight these differences.

Such discrepancies frequently have important implications for the psychiatrist's understanding of staff attitudes toward the patient.

> The psychiatrist was asked to see Mr. D., who was being treated on the neurological service for multiple sclerosis, because he was a "management problem." The patient–staff conflict seemed, at first glance, to center on the use of steroids. The patient maintained that he felt less depressed and physically stronger on steroids. However, the house staff questioned the value of this medication, and were concerned about possible side effects. Accordingly, a placebo regimen was instituted, and the consequent transient improvement in mood further convinced Mr. D.'s doctors that steroids had no beneficial effect.
>
> However, the patient's chart had numerous observations by his nurses and physical therapist in support of his contention that he felt happier and stronger on steroids. It was the task 'of the psychiatrist to make Mr. D.'s physicians aware of this pattern, which was clearly demonstrated in the chart.*

Evaluating the Nurse

Because she is in close contact with the patient for prolonged periods, the nurse can significantly enhance our understanding of the somatopsychic responses of the patient. A longitudinal view of the patient's psychological responses—for example, an evolving delirium, or the patient's response to a visit from his physician or a member of his family—may be discernible only through this source.

The psychiatrist also evaluates the nurse's relationship with the physician to ascertain the degree to which she is expected to provide psychological care for the patient. This varies from ward to ward and from service to service. And, most important, the psychiatrist evaluates the nurse's psychological-mindedness to ascertain the degree to which she can fulfill the patient's needs.

> Miss C. convinced the psychiatrist that she could deal most effectively with the needs of a male patient who was dying of a neoplasm. The patient had formed a close bond with this nurse. As a result, she was able to persuade both him and his family to verbalize their concerns about his impending death. It had been these secret feelings, which had made their being together intolerable.

> Mr. L., a Trinidadian, developed a postoperative psychosis, manifested by episodic agitation, confusion, assaultive behavior, and

---

* The psychiatrist's assessment of this patient is amplified later in this chapter.

a delusion that his penis was falling off. He refused to be seen by a psychiatrist, and would only consent to talk to his Trinidadian nurse, who was frightened by his behavior and wanted to withdraw from the case. The psychiatrist was able to help her to deal with her fears, and she demonstrated a capacity to be both firm and re-assuring to the patient. For example, she was able to say: "Take your hands off your penis. It's all right. That's only a catheter for your urine," and "Stop trying to choke me. I'm not the devil; I'm Miss A., your nurse."

In short, ideally, the nurse performs a dual function. She enhances the psychiatrist's understanding of the patient, and is an important therapeutic ally.

Evaluating the Family

If the psychiatrist feels the family's perceptions of the patient are fairly accurate, he may be able to assess the severity of the patient's psychological problem on the basis of the family's description of the patient's personality and behavior prior to the onset of his illness. For example, the psychiatrist may need to know whether the patient has always been "difficult," or fear-ful, or preoccupied with his health or physical prowess. In addition, the psychiatrist evaluates the family per se, that is, their role in the onset or exacerbation of the patient's illness and their capacity to participate in the patient's hospital and convalescent care.

Evaluating the Ward Culture

As noted earlier, routine data relevant to this aspect of the psychiatrist's inquiry are usually transmitted to the psychiatrist via the request for psy-chiatric consultation. Specifically, the psychiatrist learns whether the patient is a private or staff patient; whether he has been hospitalized for a diag-nostic work-up or for treatment of a life-threatening illness. But because there are vast differences in the medical and psychological climates of each ward, the psychiatrist must also evaluate the characteristics of the particular ward on which the patient has been placed.

Patients remain on the vascular surgery ward for one to six months. During this period, they proceed through soaks, grafts, sympathectomies, femoral bypasses, metatarsal, below-knee, and above-knee amputations, with no assurance that further surgery will not be necessary before healing is secure. The patients have little opportunity to obtain information about their condition from the surgical staff. They become increasingly angry as they wait, and since the surgeons aren't there, their anger is directed at the nurses and the "establishment." Unfortunately, although the nurses want to help, they are not able to deal with the stresses that evoke this anger.

It is essential for the psychiatrist to get a sense of the ward with regard to its patient population, nursing staff, house staff, leadership, and its philosophy of patient care. These variables—the ward culture—will influence both the psychiatrist's assessment of the patient's psychological problem and his therapeutic recommendations.

Interviewing the Patient

Because the medical patient does not come to the psychiatrist of his own volition, he may be reluctant to cooperate with the psychiatrist unless he has been prepared for the interview beforehand by his internist. Indeed, the psychiatrist should make such preparation a precondition of the consultation. Essentially, the internist should impress the patient with the fact that the psychological evaluation is an important extension of the medical work-up—that the data accumulated by the psychiatrist will help the internist to provide better treatment for his patient. The internist's ability to transmit this information in a tactful, straightforward manner often determines the success or failure of the psychiatric contact.

The goal of the interview is to provide the psychiatrist with some understanding of how the patient, with his *particular* personality and his *particular* life experience is responding, at this point in time, to his *particular* disease process and to hospitalization. The psychiatrist also needs to understand how the patient perceives the hospital staff's response to him. To gain such understanding, the psychiatrist must tap the patient's fantasies, as well as the thoughts and feelings that shape his responses and relationships with the hospital staff. These fantasies, thoughts, and feelings can usually be elicited by direct questioning: "How are they treating you here?" "Tell me about your illness, and what brought you to the hospital." "What do you know about it?" "What do you imagine is really wrong with you?" "Do you feel it's unfair that this should be happening to you, that you should have been 'chosen'?"

Life circumstances surrounding the onset of the illness, and its recurrence or exacerbation, should be explored: "When did you become ill?" "What was going on in your life at the time?" "What has made you feel better?" "When do you feel worse?" "Do you know anyone else who has had the same illness?"

Reactions that are unique to the patient should be elicited: "Everyone reacts differently to illness and hospitalization. How do you feel about being sick, having to stay in bed, and being cared for?" "What do you usually do when you're upset and nervous?" "How did you react to previous illnesses? Tell me about those illnesses." "Do you feel optimistic about your condition?" "Do you think you'll have to change your life style when you leave the hospital?" "Do you think you'll be able to adapt to a new life style?"

Although the psychiatrist does not test the patient directly, during the course of the interview he is continually assessing the patient's mental functioning. He considers such questions as: What is the patient's level of intelligence; does he understand his illness and its prognosis? Is his understanding impaired by cultural factors? Do I have to rely on his family for his past history and current life situation? Usually, the psychiatrist is able to make a fairly accurate assessment of the patient's mental capacities during the interview. Further investigation of his orientation, memory, and judgment may or may not be necessary.

The psychiatrist terminates the interview by attempting to dispel some of the patient's worrisome fantasies and correcting misinformation. He reminds the patient that he will talk with his physician, and asks him whether he has any questions. Finally, he thanks the patient for his cooperation, and tells him what further steps will be taken to alleviate his concerns.

The clinical example presented below illustrates the concept of the expanded psychiatric assessment in the medical setting.

The Request for Psychiatric Consultation

After receiving the following request from Neurology: "Please see Mr. D. because of poor adjustment and resultant depression," the psychiatric consultant contacted Mr. D.'s neurologist to discuss the problem in further detail. He learned that Mr. D. was a 34-year-old, married Hispanic who had been well until 1970, when he was hospitalized for headaches. Over the next few years he had shown progressive signs of diffuse neurological disease. In 1972, during his first admission to our hospital, a psychiatric consultation was requested to evaluate the possibility that his inability to walk had a hysterical component. A definitive diagnosis of multiple sclerosis was not made until his readmission the next month with progressive signs of muscular weakness, parasthesias, and scanning speech. The house staff had been concerned about informing Mr. D. of the diagnosis, and had delayed for several weeks. After he had been told, they noted that he read a great deal about multiple sclerosis.

Mr. D. was started on corticosteroids, but their use was erratic and finally stopped because the house staff felt the patient was trying to control the dosage by exaggerating his symptoms. Following this the patient became depressed and verbalized thoughts of suicide. In addition, he balked at physical therapy. A second psychiatric consultation was then requested.

The Doctor

The house staff's attitudes toward the patient were obvious after the consultant spoke to them. He had serious doubts about their ability and motivation to deal with Mr. D.'s psychological problems. He felt they were requesting him to take the patient off their hands, that is, to recommend his transfer to Psychiatry.

The Chart

The chart revealed that, despite the protests of the house staff, there seemed to be a correlation between the use of steroids and the description by the nurses and physical therapist of an improvement in the patient's mood and physical functioning.

The Nurse

The nurses expressed their anxiety about the patient's hyperactivity and depression. In contrast to the physicians, the nurses (and physical therapist) were overinvolved with Mr. D. and tended to baby him.

The Family

The patient's wife, who was in the final stage of pregnancy, was so distressed at the thought of her husband's being an invalid that she became significantly depressed, and stopped visiting him in the hospital. She was seriously considering divorce.

The Ward Culture

The neurological service is primarily a diagnostic-referral service, where the patient's emotional needs are secondary to organic diagnosis and management. In short, Mr. D. didn't "fit in."

The Patient*

The patient had an ingratiating quality that seemed to thinly hide a depressive mood. There was no evidence of psychosis or of an organic brain syndrome.

* Only the highlights of the interview are repeated here.

He talked spontaneously of his feelings of helplessness and fears of falling apart from his illness, and related his depression and uncertainty to his doctors' withdrawal and their ambivalent attitude about the use of steroids. It became evident that he felt he knew a great deal about his disease and wanted to have a voice in its management. A need for order, to be "in control," was a consistent theme throughout his life. Among Mr. D.'s childhood memories was a significant and extended hospitalization when he was four for an eye injury. The experience had evoked fear and a wish for his parents. He was proud of the fact that he had not "given in" to his fears, and had held back his tears.

Mr. D. viewed his illness as punishment for an extramarital affair. The illness also evoked feelings of guilt and shame because he could not live up to his father's dream that he finish graduate school. Nor could he sustain the goals his father had set for him in childhood: to be brave and physically active—a "real man." In contrast to his strong attachment to his father, as a child he had tended to push his mother away because she was always babying him and trying to keep him clean.

The interview ended on a friendly note: Mr. D. expressed the hope that his "discussion" with the psychiatrist would help other patients to cope with their illnesses.

Once the psychiatrist has accumulated sufficient information to enable an accurate formulation of the patient's psychological functioning, he is faced with the task of transmitting this knowledge in order to foster a collaborative approach that will promote its maximum utilization by the patient's various caretakers. The success of the psychiatrist's efforts to this end will depend in large measure on his ability to select for presentation those psychological and medical data that have direct relevance for the staff's understanding and management of the patient's behavior. Although this information is transmitted both verbally and in writing, it can be communicated most effectively in a verbal exchange.

In preparing his verbal presentation, the psychiatrist is guided by three considerations. First, any tendency to be authoritative or condescending will antagonize the staff. Second, the communication is formulated to arouse the staff's curiosity and interest, as well as to expand the staff's knowledge of the psychology of the medically ill, in general, and of the patient under consideration, in particular. Third, abstruse theories of the origins and dynamics of behavior and the excessive use of jargon are likely to evoke resistance in nonpsychiatric personnel.

The effective transmission—and utilization—of the diverse data on which psychiatric assessment in the liaison setting is based presupposes a thorough knowledge of the psychology of the medically ill individual, of the effects of psychological factors on the pathogenesis of medical illness, and of the effects of organic illness on psychological functioning. The remaining chapters in this section are devoted to the presentation of these concepts.

REFERENCE

1. Mendelson M, Meyer E: Psychiatric consultation on the medical and surgical wards, patterns and processes. Psychiatry 24:197–220, 1961

BIBLIOGRAPHY

Caplan G: Principles of Preventive Psychiatry. New York, Basic Books, 1964

Hackett TP, Weisman A: Psychiatric management of operative syndromes I & II. Psychosom Med 22 (4, 5)

Kimball C: Conceptual developments in psychosomatic medicine 1939–1969. Ann Intern Med 73:307–316, 1970

Lipowski ZJ: Review of consultation psychiatry and psychosomatic medicine I & II. Psychosom Med 29 (2, 3), 1967

Schiff SK, Pilot ML: An approach to psychiatric consultation in the general hospital. Arch Gen Psychiatry 1:349–357, 1959

Schwab JJ: Psychiatric Consultation. New York, Appleton-Century-Crofts, 1968

Chapter 3

Psychological Reactions to Medical Illness and Hospitalization

The intern and nurse stared wide-eyed as Mr. R., who had just been admitted to the coronary care unit for treatment of a massive coronary occlusion, ran down the hospital corridor. Nor did Mr. R.'s aberrant behavior cease after he had been chastised for his initial defiance of his doctor's orders to stay in bed. When the staff explained that bed rest was essential for his recovery, he proceeded to demonstrate his strength by lifting his bed. Even their angry warnings that he was killing himself were to no avail.

Although the staff did not pretend to understand his obstreperous behavior, Mr. R. was not at first considered a candidate for psychiatric treatment. Eventually, however, it became apparent to his doctors and nurses that some understanding of Mr. R.'s motives was essential if they were to manage this patient's life-threatening behavior. On the ninth day of Mr. R.'s hospital stay, a routine request for psychiatric consultation was placed.

The purpose of this chapter is to explain what made Mr. R run; to explain why, in fact, a significant proportion of all normal medically ill patients manifest adverse psychological reactions, of varying severity, to their illness and hospitalization that may impede their treatment and recovery. We will also discuss the management of this broad spectrum of psychological reactions.

THEORIES OF THE PSYCHOLOGY OF THE MEDICALLY ILL

Bibring and Kahana[1] are leading proponents of the view that the internist's ability to establish a character diagnosis and his knowledge of the particular traits that are associated with character types can serve as the basis for his choice of an effective approach to the psychological management of his medical patient. They have suggested, for example, that awareness of the psychological features of the oral-dependent character (e.g., the excessive dependence of such persons on the environment for supplies) would enable the internist to induce such a patient to undergo a painful diagnostic or therapeutic procedure, or to agree to be transferred to another service, by persuading him that his compliance with these required procedures will be amply rewarded. Specifically, these patients need to be assured that their "good behavior" will earn the admiration and approval (i.e., the love) of their internist. Krystal[2] has focused on the patient's typical utilization of specific defense mechanisms to ward off anxiety as the key to the understanding and management of his behavior, and has outlined a typical sequence of defensive reactions to traumatic physical illness to further demonstrate the usefulness of the approach.

We would extend Bibring and Krystal's formulations to include the concept of illness and hospitalization as a "gross" stress that mobilizes the genetic givens and psychological experiences of the total organism. All of the resources of the mental apparatus are required to master this event. Actually, the vast majority of patients are able to cope and to assume the role of patient without difficulty. And this is extraordinary in itself, when one considers the magnitude of these stresses.

The vulnerability of a given patient to such stress, and the kind of psychological response it gives rise to, will depend on many variables, including the nature of the stress he is experiencing, that is, the special meaning his illness and hospitalization hold for him; his characteristic mode of coping with stress; and his previous experiences with doctors, illness, and hospitalization.

The nature and meaning of the psychological stress evoked by the patient's illness and hospitalization and his relationship with others provide the basis for our therapeutic interventions. Consequently, we seek to understand the meaning of these stresses for the doctor as well as for the patient. Plans for the patient's effective psychological care follow naturally from such understanding. For once we are provided with this knowledge, we are able to normalize the hospital environment, and particularly the doctor–patient relationship, so that both the patient and his doctor can achieve optimal adaptation.

Basic Stresses of Illness and Hospitalization

The sick, hospitalized patient is vulnerable to seven categories of psychological stress:

1. The basic threat to narcissistic integrity.
2. Fear of strangers.

3. Separation anxiety.
4. Fear of the loss of love and approval.
5. Fear of the loss of control of developmentally achieved functions (e.g., bowel and bladder control, regulation and appropriate modulation of feeling states).
6. Fear of loss of or injury to body parts (castration anxiety).
7. Reactivation of feelings of guilt and shame, and accompanying fears of retaliation for previous transgressions.

The Basic Threat to Narcissistic Integrity.* Sudden illness, hospitalization, and the threat of death undermine the universal, albeit irrational, beliefs that we are always capable, independent, and self-sufficient; that our bodies are indestructible; that we can control the world around us and are the masters of our own destiny. These events challenge the infantile fantasy on which these beliefs are based—the fantasy that our omnipotent parents (and, later, the doctor) can ensure our pain-free, pleasurable, and protected existence. Thus, just as the child blames his parents when he hurts himself ("You should have stopped me from falling!"), the adult patient may blame the omnipotent parent-doctor for his painful illness. Similarly, the patient's belief in his autonomy and his conviction that he is "in control" of the world around him are challenged and reversed. Once he enters the hospital, the patient is expected to passively comply with myriad orders. He is told what medication to take, and when to take it; and, whether he wants to or not, he is expected to submit to a variety of diagnostic and therapeutic procedures. His activities no longer depend on his own whims and desires; they are routinized to conform with established hospital procedures. He is told when to go to sleep, when to wake up, when to eat; he may even have to go to the bathroom on schedule. In short, he is treated like an infant, but has none of the normal perquisites of the infant, for example, to behave irresponsibly, make excessive demands on those around him, or just be terribly upset.

Fear of Strangers. When the patient enters the hospital, he is expected, in a sense, to put his life in the hands of a group of strangers, to whom he has no close personal ties and who may or may not be competent to assume responsibility for his survival.

Separation Anxiety. The hospitalized patient is separated from important persons and things (e.g., his family and friends, his job, valued possessions,

---

* Normal narcissism may be defined as the emotional investment in the bodily and mental self that is manifested in feelings of well-being; that is experienced (emotionally) as a feeling of self-worth and felt (physically) as a sense of bodily integrity and strength. Feelings of confidence, self-satisfaction, and admiration of others, as well as a feeling of confidence in one's ability to achieve realistic life ambitions, are additional facets of normal narcissism.

home, and bed), culture and privacy, and an environment that provided the support and gratification that, to varying degrees, are necessary for his effective functioning and sustained sense of intactness.

The elderly patient is especially vulnerable to an unfamiliar environment. He may manifest a so-called catastrophic reaction—that is, overwhelming anxiety or depression in response to separation from his familiar environment and routine.

Fear of the Loss of Love and Approval.   Fear of the loss of love and approval may come to the fore under a variety of circumstances. The woman who has had a mastectomy may feel unattractive, undesirable—and unlovable. The driving executive who has had a heart attack, and has been ordered "to do nothing but rest," may feel that his enforced idleness will be interpreted as evidence of a decline in his physical prowess, which will result in a loss of the love of his family and the respect of his peers. The patient who suffers from a debilitating illness and requires intensive medical and nursing care may fear that his passive dependence on others may incur the disapproval of his friends and family.

Fear of the Loss of Control of Developmentally Achieved Functions.   Severe illness may undo previously mastered physical and mental functions. For example, physical strength, bowel and bladder control, motor functions, speech, and the ability to regulate one's emotions may all be interrupted temporarily. Many patients agonize over the transient loss of these basic functions to the point where despite the staff's repeated efforts to reassure them to the contrary, they remain convinced that they will never regain control of the functions.

Fear of Loss of or Injury to Body Parts.   Manifestations of castration anxiety may take various forms. Once the patient enters the hospital, his body becomes the property of his physicians, to do with what they will. His bodily fluids are drained; his body is exposed, probed, and weakened. The patient's submissive relationship to the physician and these routine hospital procedures may stir up various sexual fantasies that may include fantasies of sexual submission and penetration.

Thus, if these medical procedures are highly sexualized in the mind of the patient, he may experience them as sexual attacks on his body. By the same token, the patient who must submit to amputation may feel that the surgeon is "taking everything away from him." Castration anxiety abounds and may reach panic proportions—homosexual panic in the male, and fantasies of masochistic surrender (rape) in the female.

A 40-year-old fireman had had his pubic area shaved before undergoing an open ileac crest marrow biopsy under local anesthesia.

During the operation he overheard the following exchange between the surgeon and his assistant: "Is the incision large enough?" "No." "Do we have enough yet?" At this point, the patient yelled, "What are you taking out there?" He remained in a dissociated state for the next twenty-four hours.

A 35-year-old patient, who was impotent three months after he had undergone surgical resection for a ruptured diverticulum, showed the internist his incision and traced it from his xyphoid process to a point just above his symphisis pubis. "I think they took everything out, or cut a wire. I've been knocked out of commission. I feel dead. I wonder how much longer I'll be able to keep my wife."

Fear of the loss of body parts or functions is generated by the mechanisms of regression, symbolism, and displacement. The child of four equates real or imagined body injury with genital injury—and death. In the normal adult these fantasies remain dormant, but may be revived with medical illness.

Guilt and Fear of Retaliation.   Feelings of guilt and shame, which may be reactivated by physical illness, and the patient's fantasy that illness and hospitalization are punishment for his previous sins of omission or commission, are prominent sources of psychological stress. Thus, patients frequently berate themselves because they didn't stop smoking, or take it easy, or because their sex life was too active. And for such patients a corollary of the concept of illness as punishment is the concept of cure as forgiveness.

The fear of pain, which is also a prominent source of psychological stress, cuts across all of the categories discussed above. Each of these stresses may compound the basic painful experience; and, conversely, severe pain may increase the magnitude of each of these stresses. For example, the threat to the patient's physical integrity becomes more acute when he is in severe pain; he may view his inability to "deal" with pain as further evidence of his general loss of control of previously mastered mental functions; or his weakness in the face of pain may intensify his fear that he will lose the love and approval of important persons in his environment.

Clinical Variations of Basic Stresses

Although illness and hospitalization are inevitable sources of psychological stress for all patients, patients may not be equally vulnerable to all categories of stress. The judgment as to whether illness and hospitalization constitute a particular kind of stress for the individual patient cannot be made solely on the basis of the specific nature of these events, but requires knowledge of the patient's psychological makeup as well. For example, separation may not be experienced as a loss, but as a welcome release. A patient who longs to return to an earlier dependent state, who has strong needs to be taken care of, will not experience illness and hospitalization as a threat to his physical and emotional integrity. And another patient may have delayed seeking medical help even after his symptoms became acute, so that "the punishment would fit the crime." Or a patient may be a perpetual candidate for surgical intervention. Such patients welcome the infliction of pain, the loss of parts of their body or its functions, and even the threat of death, as just punishment for their previous transgressions— and as the means by which they can atone for these "sins."

> When the 26-year-old mother of two was told she had leukemia and might die, she reacted stoically, and calmly announced, "I knew it all the time." In her ongoing psychotherapy, begun before she was informed of this diagnosis, she described her illness as a welcome and deserved punishment for an extramarital affair that had ended long before the onset of her physical symptoms.

Other factors affecting the patient's vulnerability to stress are realistic ones—whether or not his current life style and his future goals are dramatically affected by his illness or surgery. For example, an accountant who prides himself on his "computerlike mind" may be devastated on many different levels by a stroke that leads to dyscalculia. Following a leg amputation, a young skier who had had ambitions of entering the Olympics is faced not only with castration threats but with the very real fact that he well never attain his goal.

Dynamics of Psychological Reactions to Stress

The ubiquity of these stress situations makes it possible to identify common patterns of psychological reactions among the hospitalized medical population.

Typically, patients respond to these stresses initially with a universal loss of self-esteem, which is accompanied by an unpleasant affect, or a series of unpleasant affects, such as varying degrees of "normal depression," anxiety, shame, guilt, and feelings of helplessness. If these unpleasant affects persist, or are particularly intense, the patient may replace them with inappropriate pleasant affects, with the result that he becomes euphoric or manic. Or he may attempt to cope with the stress and diminish the unpleasant affect it engenders through the use of inappropriate or unrealistic psychological mechanisms. Finally, the physiological concomitants of intense affects (e.g., anxiety and anger) may put additional strain on an already defective system (e.g., a damaged heart), and these secondary consequences may compound the psychological stress.

In general, however, we would reemphasize that the nature and magnitude of the patient's response to these stresses will depend on what illness and hospitalization mean to him in terms of his past experiences and development, and in terms of his current psychological resources. Each individual evaluates the present in terms of his past conflicts, object relationships, goals, and so forth. The stresses we have discussed parallel the stresses each individual experiences at various stages in his early development. Consequently, the patient's current ability to cope depends on whether or not he achieved adequate means of adaptation to these stresses when he experienced them as a child.

Children who were not neglected, hurt, or exposed to extreme emotional or physical traumas, whose relationship with their parents was built on trust are less likely to be threatened by a recurrence in adulthood of these stresses in the hospital setting. It is the quality of the child's relationship with his mother, in particular, that will determine the success or failure with which he adapts to the stress of illness and hospitalization in later life. However, although psychiatrists have traditionally focused on the implications of the child's relationship with his mother for his future development, in fact, the quality of his relationship with his father is important too, for it serves as a model for his future relationships with men. Ideally, the child learns from this model to be passive with a man, to trust other men, and to respond appropriately to authority without fear of losing his bodily integrity and independence (fear of being castrated).

These attitudes and feelings, which were formed early in life, and which remain underground in the compensated adult, are reactivated and intensified under the stress of illness and hospitalization, and are now directed toward the patient's medical caretakers. Very ill patients who must be fed intravenously, monitored in a coronary care unit, or undergo surgery must have achieved some early sense of trust if they are to be "successfully dependent" on the life-support ministrations of strangers.

The hospitalized patient regresses temporarily to earlier modes of behavior, when his defenses, conflicts, thinking, and relationships with others were more primitive, less discriminating, and less reality-oriented. However, regression is not pathological per se; in fact, it is normal and can enhance personal growth and mastery. Regression is an innate property of the nervous system and mental life, and it is normally activated by physical impairment or psychological stress. Consequently, like all responses to psychological and physical stress, it has both adaptive and maladaptive features. For example, if an able-bodied seaman can assume a passive-dependent role during the acute phase of his illness, if he can allow himself to be fed, bathed, and catheterized, he has regressed adaptively in the service of his recovery. If, on the other hand, the patient experiences his illness and enforced dependence on others as a threat to his physical and emotional integrity, if it evokes fear of the loss of love and fear of castration, he may need to defend against these fears by inappropriate demonstrations of his strength and virility. And, in that event, he will be unable to regress suffi-ciently to facilitate treatment and recovery. Such patients typically rely on primitive ego defenses (e.g., massive denial of their illness) and primitive modes of relating to others in an effort to maintain psychological equili-brium. On the other hand, the patient may cling to a passive-dependent role when it is no longer necessary or appropriate.

The tasks facing the patient with an acute illness differ from those facing the patient with a chronic disease. For example, the patient with an acute fulminating meningitis must deal with the realization that he suddenly has gone from feeling well, working, and loving, to being severely ill in a hospital, facing possible residual disabilities and death. This patient is usually severely anxious and may employ defenses used by people subject to other traumatic events such as fires and earthquakes; that is, he may develop a numbing depersonalization-like reaction. As the patient feels better and sees that he is "over the hump" and this is reinforced by the physician's reassurance, his use of primitive mechanisms lessens and he becomes less dependent and more of an ally to his idealized doctor. Improvement serves as a built-in positive reinforcement. The doctor feels intellectually chal-lenged by the acute disease, and he feels optimistic because of his potent therapeutic armamentarium, and this attitude is imparted to the patient who, in turn, bolsters the doctor's self-esteem.

The patient with chronic illness, such as diabetes, especially the juvenile type, is faced with different stresses. On the positive side, the duration of the illness allows for the development of defenses to deal with anxiety and for the adaptation to a disease-compatible life style. However, this psy-chological adaptation is undermined when his symptoms worsen; when he goes into a coma or shock reaction; when long-term complications such as blindness and vascular reactions occur; and when he must face the inevita-bility of a shorter life span. At such times his defenses must shift. Long-term denial is broken down, and he may lose faith in his doctors, become depressed, and doctor-shop. Unlike the patient with an acute illness, this patient cannot see day-to-day improvement. On the contrary, he may see progressive deterioration. The physician cannot realistically say he's getting better. Instead, he might have to bolster the patient by reassuring him about how well he is coping with such a difficult situation. The doctor's relation-ship with the patient is much more primitive; for example, he must con-stantly reassure the patient verbally and in action that he will not abandon him.

Stresses on the Physician

Understanding of the doctor–patient relationship hinges on recognition of the role of stress as an inherent feature of human growth and maturation. In the course of his own emotional development, the internist has been exposed to the same conflicts as his patient, and he brings these unresolved (albeit quiescent) conflicts to the clinical setting. The patient's attitudes and behavior, and the nature and outcome of the illness, may revive these conflicts in his medical caretakers. And, as is true of the patient, the internist's vulnerability to the patient's reaction to stress will depend on the quality of his object relationships, past and present, and the degree to which he has resolved his own childhood conflicts. For example, the patient who doesn't get better may threaten the doctor's sense of narcissistic integrity. Contact with new patients and their families may revive the internist's strong feelings of stranger anxiety. Medical caretakers may react adversely when they are not loved or admired by their patients (even as they may resent being cast in the role of all-caring, all-accepting parent). They may identify with patients who must undergo mutilating procedures, and experience the same degree of stress. And, as might be expected, the dying patient frequently evokes feelings of guilt and shame in his medical caretakers, who berate themselves for not keeping an adequate vigil or for not knowing enough about the illness to help the patient.

Thus, the internist is charged with a dual responsibility. Clearly, if he is to provide adequate medical and psychological care for his patient, he must understand the nature of the psychological stresses provoked in the patient by his illness and hospitalization, and be able to help him to cope with these stresses. But he must also possess sufficient self-knowledge to recognize and cope with the stresses under which he is operating. Otherwise these stresses may adversely affect his relationship with and attitudes toward the patient, with the result that he may become either too involved with or too remote from the patient.

The internist's problem is further compounded by the fact that the posture he assumes in his interactions with the patient (and the patient's attitudes toward his caretakers) does not remain static. The sequence of becoming ill, being treated, and then recovering implies a constantly changing doctor–patient relationship. Each stage has its own stresses. The patient who has just suffered a myocardial infarction must remain completely passive during the initial, critical stage of his illness. As the patient recovers, his autonomous activities increase in extent and power. Similarly, the surgical patient is considered a "good" patient if he is able to remain quiet and follow orders for the first few hours immediately following his operation. At this stage it is most important that he be able to regress sufficiently to assume a completely dependent role. Later on, however, the patient's role changes. Once he has recovered from the initial trauma of surgery, the patient must try to sit up, walk, and cough against pain, if he is to be regarded as a "good" patient. Actually, this transition from passivity to activity, from total dependence to relative independence, may take place in just a few hours, but it signals the beginning of physiological and psychological recovery. The doctor plays a crucial role in the implementation of these adaptive changes in the patient's behavior and attitudes. He must be flexible to achieve a delicate balance, catering to the patient's dependency needs even as he encourages independence. But, most important, medical caretakers must be sufficiently flexible to accept the fact that their patients may not always be able to fulfill the prerequisites of the "good" patient or to adhere to a proscribed timetable in making the transition from passivity to activity.

Within this conceptual framework we have found it useful to evaluate the doctor–patient relationship in terms of three interrelated dynamic "systems":

1. The stage of the patient's illness (or convalescence).
2. The patient's personal reaction to his illness and to his internist.
3. The internist's reaction to his patient and to his patient's illness.

The goal of the psychiatrist is to detect discordance in these systems. Any one, or all three, may be out of phase, producing an angry, disruptive patient, or an anxious, withdrawn doctor.

> A 75-year-old man who had suffered a stroke, but had recovered sufficient motor capacity for limited self-care, was extremely angry with the resident because he hadn't been washed and fed. The patient's behavior evoked a counterdefensive reaction in the resident, who challenged him by saying, "Do more for yourself," after which he turned his back and abruptly walked away. To make matters worse, on his way out he murmured an aside to a colleague (which was overheard by the patient) to the effect that he couldn't stand patients like that. After this episode, the patient said, "I wish I were dead."

The doctor's response to this patient was out of phase with the stage of the patient's illness and its meaning for him. The patient's needs (which, admittedly, were somewhat unrealistic), as well as his resultant anger, should have been understood as an attempt to compensate for his feelings of being damaged and helpless, and they should have been dealt with directly. Instead, and inevitably, this confrontation produced feelings of guilt and shame in doctor and patient alike. The patient's stated wish that he would die seemed to stem from his feelings of mortification and guilt, and, of course, it was also an attempt to punish his doctor. But, perhaps because of the staff's own guilt, the patient's statement was interpreted by them as evidence of his suicidal tendencies, and a request for a psychiatric consultation was promptly initiated.

CLINICAL CORRELATIONS

A synthesis of the material presented above enables the construction of criteria to assess the patient's capacity to adapt to the hospital experience and the extent to which the doctor has contributed to or detracted from that capacity for adaptation. Treatment is based on an evaluation of the patient, in terms of his psychological response to the stress of illness and hospitalization, and on an assessment of the doctor–patient relationship in terms of the three dynamic systems cited earlier. Obviously, however, if treatment is to be effective, other factors must also be taken into account. Our treatment plan must take into consideration the culture of the medical setting, including a realistic assessment of the working time available to psychiatric and ward personnel for such purposes; the capacity of the house staff for self-understanding, as well as the degree to which they are capable of understanding and dealing with the patient's psychological problem; and, finally, the medical and psychological status of the particular patient in need of the services of the psychiatrist. Above all, our therapeutic approach is a dynamic one that is flexible enough to incorporate changes in the patient's psychological status, in the disease process, and in the patient's medical management.

Given this orientation, the prerequisites for successful adaptation to illness and hospitalization include:

1. The patient's ability to regress adequately in the service of recovery.
2. His ability to maintain adequate defenses against the stresses evoked by illness and hospitalization.
3. Access to his feelings and fantasies, and the ability to communicate his needs.
4. A basic trust in his medical caretakers.
5. The services of empathic and flexible physicians and nurses.

Case Illustration

Mr. R., the patient described earlier, who had just suffered a major heart attack, deliberately disregarded his internist's orders to remain in bed (and, instead, tried to lift the bed to demonstrate his strength), ran up and down the hospital corridors, and so forth. Nine days later, when it became clear that his doctors and nurses could do nothing to control his life-threatening agitation, they agreed that the patient's psychological management was the most urgent issue. Up to this point, although the staff had recognized that Mr. R.'s behavior was bizarre, they hadn't known what to do about it. Consequently, they handled it by neglect. Presumably, they hoped his behavior would improve with time.

The data accumulated by the psychiatrist in the course of his interview with Mr. R.—particularly the history of early defiance, of his need to prove his manhood because of his strong latent homosexual feelings, and of his marked depression and agitation on previous hospitalizations—enabled him to understand the patient's current behavior. Moreover, these data allowed him to build a rational approach to Mr. R.'s irrational behavior within the conceptual framework described above, that is, the five elements necessary for successful adaptation to illness and hospitalization:

Adequate Regression

The key issue was how to facilitate adequate regression so that Mr. R. would become a "good" patient. As a child, he would only do what he was told to do if his mother cried and pleaded with him. We attempted to manipulate his environment by getting his wife to beg him to stay in bed "for her," and it worked. The nurses, physical therapist, and attendants all approached him in this manner.

We also appealed to his phallic narcissism, and used it as a vehicle to facilitate regression, that is, to allow himself to be cared for: "It takes quite a man to be able to stay in bed! You must have a lot of patience to do those toe and finger exercises so persistently. You're such a well-built guy, let's stick to that diet." Mr. R. was then able to permit himself to give in a little and still maintain his self-esteem.

Adequate Defenses

We fostered his intellectual defenses by letting him tell us about coronary disease, and by providing him with whatever factual data he wanted (as evidence of our respect for his intelligence). Because he felt that we admired (and needed) him more than he admired or needed us, Mr. R. could deny his intolerable fear of becoming dependent.

The toe and finger exercises enabled the motor discharge of tension, which increased the patient's ability to tolerate anxiety, made him less prone to self-destructive action, and less likely to use primitive defenses, such as paranoid projection. Our efforts in these areas were further facilitated by the use of tranquilizers and hypnotics, which reduced anxiety and fatigue, with the result that Mr. R. felt more in control. At the same time, as his anxiety diminished, his ability to put his feelings into words increased, making him more accessible to hospital management.

Access to Feelings and Fantasies, and Ability to Communicate Needs

In the face of his doctors' verbal threats, Mr. R. became more defensive and mistrustful and increasingly hyperactive. However, once they stopped telling him he would die if he didn't stay in bed, he was able to talk about the way he felt. Specifically, he described his fantasy that his heart attack was a punishment for engaging in intense sexual activity the preceding night. And he ventilated his bizarre theory that his heart would stop if he stopped being hyperactive. Mr. R.'s hyperactivity stemmed from his fantasy that he had to "keep his motor going"—that he had a "switch" inside him, and once this "switch" was turned off, it could never be turned on again. When this fantasy had been dealt with and dispelled (through reality testing), Mr. R.'s doctors were able to empathize with his more realistic anxieties, and this allowed him to talk more and react less.

Basic Trust

Mr. R. began to develop a feeling of basic trust in his medical caretakers when he realized that his physicians were no longer threatening him. He found they would listen to and respect his needs, and that they helped to reduce his anxiety.

Empathic and Flexible Physicians and Nurses

When the house staff understood the historical and current issues that motivated Mr. R.'s behavior, they became more flexible. They could then respect his life style, and were able to adapt hospital routine to conform with that life style. For example, they were able to relax the rigid rules governing visits by the family; Mr. R.'s wife was permitted to bring him his favorite foods; and he was allowed to choose the arm from which blood was drawn. Furthermore, nurses were used whenever possible to mitigate Mr. R.'s fear of men. Once these measures were instituted, it was no longer necessary for Mr. R. to attempt to exercise control through defiant or destructive behavior.

However inconsequential these interventions may appear on the surface, the fact is that they enabled Mr. R. to make a satisfactory recovery from a major coronary attack.

REFERENCES

1. Bibring G, Kahana R: Lectures in Medical Psychology. New York, International Universities Press, 1968
2. Krystal H (ed): Massive Psychic Trauma. New York, International Universities Press, 1969, pp. 277–296

BIBLIOGRAPHY

Bergman A: Children in the Hospital. New York, International Universities Press, 1966

Freud A: The role of bodily illness in the mental life of children. PSA Study of the Child, Vol VII. New York, International Universities Press, 1952, pp. 69–81

Freud S: On narcissism, an introduction. In Standard Edition of the Complete Psychological Works of Sigmund Freud, Vol 14. London, Hogarth, 1957, pp. 67–102

Freud S: Inhibitions, symptoms and anxiety. In Standard Edition of the Complete Psychological Works of Sigmund Freud, Vol 20. London, Hogarth, 1959, pp. 77–175

Kohut H: The Analysis of the Self. New York, International Universities Press, 1971

Mahler M: On Human Symbiosis and the Viscissitudes of Individuation. New York, International Universities Press, 1968

Nunberg H: Practice and theory of psychoanalysis. Nerv Ment Dis, Monograph Series # 74:174, 1948

Chapter 4

Organic Precipitants of Psychological Dysfunction

Up to this point, our discussion of the etiology, diagnosis, and management of psychological dysfunction in the medically ill has been limited to patients whose symptoms arise in response to psychological stress evoked by illness and hospitalization. In this chapter we turn our attention to those patients who manifest certain distinctive mental symptoms as a consequence of pathological physical processes that, by virtue of their effect on the structure or metabolism of the brain, produce the organic brain syndromes. We discuss the organic brain syndromes from two perspectives: first, in terms of the problem these syndromes present for both the internist and the psychiatrist, and, second, in terms of their clinical features, diagnosis, and treatment.

THE PROBLEM

Given the relationship between somatic and psychic factors, which is intrinsic to the organic brain syndromes, their course and outcome depends on the ability of the patient's caretakers to function effectively in both the physiological and psychological spheres. Unfortunately, however, neither the internist nor the psychiatrist is competent to assume total responsibility for the physiological and psychological care of this patient population. The internist is not always able to diagnose an organic brain syndrome. Yet, such a diagnosis, followed by effective treatment, is often lifesaving, or, at least, can enable the patient to make maximal use of his remaining faculties. Even when the organic brain syndrome is recognized, the internist has little interest in further diagnosis or treatment, and depends on the psychiatrist to assume responsibility for the patient. The psychiatrist can detect the presence of an organic brain syndrome—provided the internist recognizes the need for his services. But the psychiatrist is not equipped to perform the necessary medical work-up and to carry out medical management; nor can he always recommend appropriate medical procedures. One would think, therefore, that the organic brain syndromes would be an ideal meeting ground for medicine and psychiatry, providing a unique opportunity to exchange ideas and evolve a team approach to diagnosis and treatment. In fact, the organic brain syndromes can serve as a model for the holistic approach. Instead, there is an inclination on the part of workers in both disciplines to abdicate responsibility for the care of these patients.

In part, the internist's difficulties stem from the characteristics of this patient population. Some patients manage to conceal their mental defects, so that they are only apparent on direct, specific examination. The internist may not regard apathy, sleepiness, weakness, or excessive fatigue as indicative of the possible presence of an organic syndrome. And, obviously, if he doesn't regard these symptoms as significant and attempt further examination of the patient, he is not likely to request a psychiatric consultation to establish a definitive diagnosis.

Other patients manifest behavior so deranged that it is frightening to the internist and psychiatrist alike. These patients are profoundly disturbed, showing diffuse anxiety, agitation, and bizarre mental and motor behavior. The internist does not hesitate to request a psychiatric consultation in such cases, but his aim is to press for the patient's transfer to the psychiatric service.

A third group of patients manifest, to varying degrees, the psychological and behavioral disturbances that characterize patients in the first two categories. If the patient is confused, disoriented, forgetful—and elderly—the internist may, without further attempts at diagnosis, automatically ascribe his behavior to the presence of degenerative brain disease and initiate plans for his disposition. Or, if the patient is younger, the internist may interpret his behavioral disturbance as evidence of a functional disorder, and a request for psychiatric treatment will be initiated.

Since the presence of an organic brain syndrome can be detected easily in the majority of cases, ideally the internist should be able to make this diagnosis. The inability of many internists to do so can only be explained on a deeper level. Because they work within a physical frame of reference, internists can use physical methods such as brain scan and x-ray to study certain aspects of brain functioning. However, using quantitative methods for measuring brain output, that is, the patient's capacity to verbalize, symbolize, remember, make appropriate judgments, engage in abstract thought, synthesize, is not part of the internist's modus operandi.[1]

But this physical orientation of the internist's training cannot adequately explain his reluctance to undertake the routine task of assessing the patient's mental functioning. Other factors may reinforce his avoidance of this area.

The task itself may give rise to one of several reactions in the internist: a fear of hurting the patient, or a wish to hurt him; a fear of embarrassing the patient, or a wish to embarrass him. These reactions are evoked when the patient's predicament touches on the internist's inner fears that his own mental limitations will some day be exposed. Therefore, often the internist does not inquire into this sector of the patient's mental functioning. His examination lacks depth, breadth, and sufficient specificity to elicit compensated deficits because of his need to protect the patient—and himself —against exposure of these deficits.

The internist's failure to provide these patients with adequate medical care can also be attributed to his failure to fully understand the pathophysiology of diseases that may impair cerebral functioning. To illustrate, as a general rule, the internist views delirium tremens as a disorder, due in most cases to the excessive ingestion of alcohol, which responds to medical treatment. He is not likely to conceptualize the syndrome in more comprehensive terms, that is, in terms of the dynamic pathophysiological effects of alcohol on the central nervous and vascular systems. For example, alcohol may affect the level of consciousness, the frontal lobe, the brain stem, the cerebellum, the spinal column, the peripheral nerves (interpretation of sensory input and motor behavior), and the integrity of blood vessels (fragility), and their sequelae make the patient more vulnerable to falls and trauma. The medical complications of delirium tremens, for example, dehydration, pneumonia, cardiovascular stress, are approached with vigor and enthusiasm, because the doctor regards them as life-threatening. Yet, they do not pose a greater danger to life than does damage to the frontal lobes, for example, which commonly produces a confused, delusional, hallucinatory state that may precipitate violent irrational behavior, including attempts at suicide. Unfortunately, these somatopsychic phenomena do not arouse the internist's interest. After the medical complications of delirium tremens have been treated, the patient is viewed as a psychiatric problem by the house staff, who are thereby deprived of the excitement of understanding the pathophysiological and pathopsychological processes that underlie their patient's extraordinary behavior.

CLINICAL FEATURES OF THE ORGANIC BRAIN SYNDROMES

Two clinical features of the organic brain syndromes that are frequently overlooked in contemporary medical practice should be emphasized at the outset. One, a variety of diverse disease entities, involving widely disparate pathological processes, may be implicated in the etiology of the organic brain syndromes. Two, contrary to popular belief, the organic brain syndromes are not necessarily irreversible. For general purposes of diagnostic classification, they can be divided into two major categories: Transient disturbances of cerebral metabolism produce acute, reversible syndromes that are referred to as "delirium." Disturbances in which structural damage occurs and neurons are destroyed produce chronic and irreversible syndromes that are referred to as "dementia." The same etiological agent may produce temporary or permanent brain damage.

Engel[2] has estimated that 10 to 15 percent of all patients hospitalized on acute medical and surgical services manifest an acute organic brain syndrome (delirium) of varying severity. Delirium is present in every patient who is approaching or recovering from coma, who is terminal, who is recovering from general anesthesia, or who is drugged to the point of confusion. It is present in most patients with severe anemia, fever, peripheral circulatory collapse, cardiac arrest, congestive heart failure, respiratory failure, pulmonary insufficiency, hepatic or renal insufficiency, acidosis or alkalosis, electrolyte imbalance, or infection. It is also present in those suffering from the effects of many different drugs, and from the effects on the central nervous system of almost every disease that produces a disturbance in physiological homeostasis.

In short, the organic brain syndromes are among the psychological disorders most frequently encountered in the contemporary teaching hospital. And they are also the most undertreated. Simon and Kahan's study[3] in 1963 of the elderly chronically ill medical population in a San Francisco hospital yielded the finding that in 50 percent of the subjects studied the presence of an acute organic syndrome, superimposed upon their chronic syndrome, and produced by vitamin deficiency, dehydration, and other factors, had not been detected—or treated. And Engel makes the point that it is impossible to estimate how many patients who suffer from acute reversible brain syndromes (delirium) at the outset subsequently develop irreversible brain damage (dementia) because the underlying organic defect remained uncorrected for too long a period.

Despite medical evidence to the contrary, there is a persistent tendency among internists to regard both dementia and delirium as "hopeless." It is true that many patients with organic brain syndromes are aged, without families, and often express the wish to die. Often these syndromes accompany terminal illness, which reinforces the tendency of the medical staff to view them as "end states," and disposition problems. But the association of the organic mental syndromes with the aged and dying fails to differentiate between acute (reversible) and chronic (irreversible) syndromes. And it does not take into account the fact that either type of organic brain syndrome can occur at any age.

Regardless of the nature of the pathological process which precipitated the organic brain syndrome, and regardless of whether that syndrome is reversible or irreversible, the physical stresses which damage the structure of the higher centers of the brain or interfere with cerebral metabolism characteristically produce deficits in the patient's mental functioning.

The nature of these deficits gain clarity when they are viewed within the conceptual framework of ego psychology. Considered within this framework the only clinical feature may be the patient's subjective feeling that he is not himself. Or physical stresses that interfere with brain function may alter a host of ego functions, for example, orientation, memory, intellectual capacity, judgment, stability of mood, impulse control, defenses, perception, motor control, level of consciousness, and attention. Additional ego functions—relationship to reality, object relationships, concept formation, and synthetic function, among others—may be affected as well, to varying degrees.

Furthermore, regression may take place, allowing for a more primitive moral and ethical code (impairment of superego functions); and there may be a breakthrough of heretofore-repressed sexual and aggressive impulses. Freud,[4] who postulated the existence of a hierarchy of mental functioning and regression based on the physiological model suggested by Hughlings Jackson, hypothesized that the functions that were most complex, and had developed last, would be the most vulnerable to early disruption, while the more primitive functions would be the most enduring.

The way in which the patient copes with these deficits in mental functioning will depend on the nature and course of the illness that precipitated the organic brain syndrome, the nature and severity of the deficits produced by the syndrome, and the patient's premorbid character style and personality. A further determinant of the patient's coping ability is the speed with which the lesion develops. When the onset of an organic lesion is acute, the patient is given very little time to make a gradual adjustment to the mental defects produced by the lesion. In contrast, slowly developing (chronic) lesions enable gradual adaptation. Consequently, although the patient with a chronic brain syndrome may sustain enormous deficits in mental functioning, he may be better able to deal with them. On the other hand, when the onset of the lesion is rapid, and there has not been sufficient time for a defensive adaptation to occur, the patient may be vulnerable to a "catastrophic reaction,"[5] that is, a disorderly, defective performance, with anxiety, agitation, irritability, and/or depression. For example, the patient, and particularly the elderly patient, whose mental capacities are impaired is more likely to react adversely to the stresses of illness and hospitalization. Adaptation requires mental tasks that he cannot perform. Consequently, these patients may develop a catastrophic reaction when they are exposed to an alien environment, expected to relate to strangers, or to adjust to new routines.

In summary, there is a constant interaction between the organic dysfunction and the patient's psychological functioning (which reflect his conflicts and personality structure). But, in addition, both of these processes —the organic and the psychological—may adversely affect the patient's physiological status, and vice versa. For example, a bout of congestive heart failure may cause an organic brain syndrome which will adversely affect the patient's psychological functioning. Psychological symptoms (anxiety, agitation, hyperkinetic motor discharge) may then produce further impairment of cardiac function, which, in turn, will worsen his organic brain syndrome. And if this vicious circle is not interrupted, this sequence of events may have a fatal outcome.

The clinical features of the organic brain syndrome may precipitate yet another vicious circle if it results in the patient's inability to form an adaptive alliance with his doctor and nurse which would allow him to become their "natural ally" in the pursuit of health. The patient's inability to attend to the doctor's directions, to remember the nurse's instructions, to cooperate in medical procedures, to acknowledge attempts by the doctor and nurse to be helpful, may evoke resentment in his caretakers, especially if they do not recognize that the patient's negative behaviors can be ascribed to an organic brain syndrome.

DIAGNOSIS

The mental status of the normal medical patient can be assessed from one of two apparently divergent positions: the neurological–psychological viewpoint (the mental status examination), or the psychoanalytic viewpoint (assessment of ego functions). What is not generally recognized is the fact that these approaches can, and sometimes must, complement and supplement each other. Both examine mental functioning, but proceed along different paths. And in using a single methodological approach, information which may be critical to this task is overlooked.

The mental status examination does not lend itself to conceptualization of the patient's performance in terms of the broader issue of his overall functioning. For example, if the extent of the patient's deficit is to be understood, and if he is to be treated effectively, we need to know what the deficit means in terms of his ability to adapt to his illness and hospitalization. If he relies solely on the mental status examination, the examiner will deduce from the patient's inability to perform—for example, to do serial 7's, draw a person—that he has a lesion in the brain, but he does not tend to translate his findings on the patient's cognitive deficit into clinical terms. Given his training in ego psychology, one would expect the psychiatrist to recognize that an evaluation of the patient's ego functions would extend the range of his observations beyond the data derived from the classic mental status examination. Instead, the mental status examination currently constitutes the psychiatrist's primary diagnostic tool. Furthermore, the psychiatrist does not fully understand the significance of the findings derived therefrom.

Both these approaches to the assessment of mental functioning are illustrated below in order to dramatize their connecting links.

PSYCHOANALYTIC TRIPARTITE MODEL OF MENTAL FUNCTIONING*

Ego Functions	*Dysfunction*
Perception	Illusions, hallucinations
Capacity to attend	Patient is distracted, with decreased concentration
Orientation	Impaired
Memory	Impaired
Comprehension	Impaired
Capacity for abstract thought	Concretization
Ability to synthesize	Impaired
Adaptation	Patient is inflexible, rigid
Defensive functions	Use of primitive and rigid defenses
Motor expression	Poorly controlled
Language	Compromise of syntax, concretization, primary process
Object relations	Regressive; unfamiliar objects become familiar through misperception, and vice versa
Mood	Labile; anxious, agitated, depressed, euphoric
Sense of integrity	Patient doesn't feel like old self
Intellectual capacity	Impaired
Judgment	Impaired

Superego Functions	*Dysfunction*
Conscience—capacity for critical evaluation	Deterioration of moral code
Self-esteem regulation	Labile, with tendency toward self-deprecation and feelings of humiliation

Id Functions†	*Dysfunction*
Aggressive drive ⎱ Expression	Hyperaggressive, hypoaggressive behavior (anergic states); agitation, restlessness, impulsivity
Sexual drive ⎰	Hypersexuality, hyposexuality

* This schema has been adapted for the assessment of the organic mental patient seen on the medical ward. The list of ego, superego, and id functions is selective, and would not lend itself to an assessment of the patient's total personality.

† These drives press for discharge, but are never seen in pure form. In the organically intact patient only the derivatives of drives are seen, after they have been shaped and regulated by the ego and superego. In the patient with an organic brain syndrome they may be expressed more directly. (It is well known, for example, that dangerous aggressive outbursts may follow temporal lobe epileptic attacks.)

MENTAL STATUS EXAMINATION*

General Information

1. Level of consciousness: alert; lethargic; stuperous; stable; fluctuating
2. Cooperation: good; fair; poor
3. Reliability of information provided
4. Motor status: posture
5. Affect: appropriate—inappropriate; euphoric—depressed; labile—flat
6. Language: expression; comprehension; coherence; voice quality (pitch, intensity, rate of speech, etc.); relevance; productivity; deviations
7. Patterns of thought: depressive; obsessive; paranoid; hypochondriacal; evidence of presence of illusions, hallucinations, delusions

Specific Information

1. Orientation
   Time
   Place
   Person
2. Insight
   e.g., Why are you in the hospital? What is the matter with you? Who am I?
3. Remote memory (storage—retrieval)
   Previously learned material
   e.g., days of the week; months of the year; patient's birthday and place of birth
   Naming visual stimuli
   e.g., colors; objects; shapes
   General fund of information
   e.g., Who is the president of the United States, the governor of the state, the mayor of the city?
4. Recent memory (registration—storage and retrieval)
   General information
   e.g., How did you get to the hospital? What did you eat for breakfast?
   Immediate recall
   Digit span: The patient is given a series of numbers by the examiner, and asked to repeat them forward and backward.
   Delayed recall
   e.g., Three items are read to the patient, who is asked to repeat them five minutes later.
5. Calculation
   e.g., The patient is asked to do simple arithmetic problems, serial 7's.
6. Abstract thinking
   Similarities
   e.g., How are a pear and an apple alike?
   Differences
   e.g., What is the difference between a lie and a mistake?
   Proverb interpretation
   e.g., What does "A bird in the hand is worth two in the bush" mean?

---

* Adapted from the mental status examination presently used at Montefiore Hospital and Medical Center (Form #MR–684). Obviously, the mental status examination is not inclusive. It is intended to serve as a "mock-up," and is provided solely for purposes of comparison with the tripartite model of mental functioning.

7. Judgment

> e.g., What would you do if you found a stamped, addressed envelope in the street?

8. Other frequently given tasks

> Writing
>
> Spatial organization (match design, map drawing, etc.)
>
> Drawing (e.g., figure copying; patient is asked to draw a clock, a daisy, etc.)
>
> Body image (e.g., patient is asked to draw a person; identification of body parts)

It is generally recognized that the conventional mental status examination, which, as noted above, is the primary diagnostic tool in the organic brain syndromes, may not be sufficiently sensitive to its task. In recent years several workers have identified defects in the standard mental status examination and developed more refined techniques to measure mental functioning. For example, Talland[6] found that even patients with severe Korsakoff's psychosis performed adequately on the part of the examination designed to test memory by requiring the patient to repeat a series of digits forward (digit span). Schwartz[7] has developed a delayed recall and interposed task which has significantly enhanced the discriminatory diagnostic power of the routine digit span test. Some workers have tried to develop more sensitive measures.*

Concretization of thought is one of the most frequent results of brain damage or cortical dysfunction. Mattis[8] strongly recommends the use of categorization tasks, such as those included in the WAIS (Wechsler Adult Intelligence Scale) Similarities Subtest. He feels that these tasks, which are relatively insensitive to disturbance due to psychogenic factors, may be the most valid measures of concrete thinking. The characteristic response of the brain-damaged patient to the WAIS Similarities Subtest question, "How are a dog and a lion alike?" is, "They are not alike. A dog is a dog, and a lion is a lion. One is tame and the other is wild. They are not the same at all."[9] Further discrimination can be achieved via the Mattis Dementia Rating Scale.[8] Here the patient is asked to name three things in a specific category, for example, what people eat. Most patients with an organic brain syndrome can offer three items, such as "hamburgers, frankfurters, and baked beans." But they are unable to give the name of the category to which these items belong. Mattis infers from such a response that the patient's deductive reasoning is relatively intact, but inductive reasoning (abstraction) is no longer available.

Finally, at times the mental status examination may not be sufficiently

---

* One attempt to develop an abbreviated, reliable mental status examination is the Mini Mental Status Exam by S. Folstein, M. Folstein, and P. R. McHugh, which is scheduled for publication in the near future (Psych Res, in press). A second effort by Jacobs, Schwartz, Delgado, and Strain to enable the rapid reliable assessment of the mental status of the hospitalized medical patient is currently in work at Montefiore Hospital and Medical Center.

sensitive for differential diagnosis. On the one hand, depression, anxiety, catastrophic reactions, and so on, are frequently encountered in the brain-damaged patient. On the other hand, short-term memory can be seriously disrupted in an organically intact patient by anxiety, depression, intrusive ideation, and idiosyncratic associative thinking.[8] Thus the task of differentiating between a functional disorder and an organic brain syndrome may pose a diagnostic dilemma in such cases which may defy immediate solution.

Other variables, in addition to the affects mentioned above, may contaminate test findings. At times, patients are so afraid the examiner will think they're crazy that they try to conceal their symptoms from him. In such instances, even the most tactfully posed question may offend and humiliate the patient. If he gets the impression from the content of a question that the examiner thinks he's crazy, or that he's stupid or uneducated, his responses to subsequent questions may be guarded or incomplete. On the other hand, a patient may not volunteer the information that she has olfactory hallucinations not because she wants to conceal the fact, but because they have "become part" of her.

In addition, the examiner must bear in mind that organicity presents a fluctuating picture in both the acute and chronic syndromes. Changes occur from moment to moment, from day to day, and gradual changes occur over weeks or months. Shands,[10] who has described the development of psychological and behavioral symptoms in the organic patient, has emphasized the importance of serial evaluations of the patient's mental status.

In some instances, the findings derived from the mental status examination may be the only clue to the presence of an on-going physical illness.

> Mr. F., a 64-year-old crane operator, was admitted to the hospital's medical service for renal shutdown, secondary to systemic lupus erythematosis. Steroids were administered to control the primary disease, and he was given dialysis to correct the biochemical disturbances associated with the extensive kidney involvement. He was discharged from the hospital on a reduced dose of steroids.
>
> Two weeks later, Mr. F. was readmitted with new somatic complaints, among them, numbness in his legs. According to the medical resident, there was no evidence that a change had occurred in his medical status. However, the resident reported that the patient appeared "confused." His wife complained that he had become increasingly "difficult" at home, and the patient admitted that he had not returned to work for fear he might kill someone with his crane. He also told the resident that he had bought two cars since his previous hospitalization. The resident concluded that the patient was in remission medically, but was suffering from a primary functional psychiatric disorder.

Psychiatric examination revealed that Mr. F.'s decision to buy two cars, which had so impressed the resident, had been made some time before he became ill, and that these purchases were appropriate. However, the patient was clearly suffering from an organic brain syndrome—as evidenced by his inability to calculate, to remember items after five minutes, and to exercise sound judgment.

One of three factors might have been implicated in the etiology of Mr. F.'s organic brain syndrome: a steroid "psychosis," cerebral involvement from systemic lupus erythematosis, or a return of renal impairment with secondary metabolic disturbance. Further medical tests revealed that the patient's renal function had indeed worsened, and an increase in steroids was instituted. Mr. F.'s psychological symptoms were the first sign of his deteriorating medical condition. It is apparent that a mental status examination must be supplemented by an assessment of ego functions for accurate diagnosis. This combined assessment of the patient provides guidelines for optimal treatment.

THE TREATMENT PLAN

Treatment of the organic brain syndromes requires a two-pronged approach: the patient's organic dysfunction requires prompt intervention, where feasible; and the psychological and behavioral aspects of the dysfunction require psychological intervention, where feasible.

In most cases, the doctor's decision as to the main thrust of treatment will be determined by individual patient considerations. Obviously, it is essential that extremely agitated patients be offered immediate symptomatic relief. This can be accomplished by the use of psychotropic drugs (see Chap. 9). However, the precipitous use of sedatives may confuse the clinical picture, or even contribute to the severity of the brain syndrome. For example, sedatives may alter the state of consciousness, and thereby obscure the diagnosis and course of a subdural hematoma. On the other hand, there are times when the patient's behavior must be controlled immediately, by whatever means available, as a lifesaving measure.

> When Mr. M., 43 years old, was admitted to the emergency room for treatment of delirium tremens, he was febrile, tachypnic, diaphoretic, and had a tachycardia of 120. In addition, he was hallucinatory, extremely anxious, and so combative that he had to be physically restrained. Because of a recent myocardial infarction, Mr. M.'s behavior was considered life-threatening, and it had to be altered immediately.

In other cases, treatment of the cause of an organic syndrome has first priority. For it is safe to assume that the psychological sequelae of the patient's organic dysfunction will remit once his organic integrity has been restored.

> Mrs. T. had been sent to the hospital's emergency room by her private internist with a diagnosis of schizophrenia. The patient's orientation, memory, and judgment were impaired, and she talked in a gibberish reminiscent of the "word salad," which is a cardinal symptom of schizophrenia.
>
> But it was the psychiatrist's impression that Mrs. T., who had lost sixty pounds over an eight-month period, was physically ill. She looked dehydrated and was febrile. Blood studies showed that she had a hemacrit of 41, a normal WBC, a sodium of 105, and chloride of 69.
>
> Within twenty-four hours after fluid and electrolyte replacement were begun, the patient was alert and oriented.

For obvious reasons, it would not have been feasible to attempt to correct the massive psychological regression, castration fears, dependency conflicts, and sadistic fantasies which were prominent features of Mrs. T.'s psychosis. Instead treatment focused on the modification of her underlying organic deficit in the expectation that this intervention would cure her disorder.

When the patient's organic dysfunction is irreversible, ideally, the internist should also be able to provide psychological treatment which will maximize his remaining resources. When the internist is unable to provide such treatment, as a consequence of defects in his medical training, he relies upon the psychiatrist to assume this responsibility. However, the psychiatrist, too, may be limited in this regard. Although he is able to alleviate the patient's acute symptomatology, by and large, the psychiatrist neglects the patient's long-term psychological needs. He makes no effort to help the patient to adapt to his organic deficits, to use his intact capacities to compensate for other losses; nor does the psychiatrist attempt to manipulate the patient's environment, or enlist the cooperation of his family in achieving these treatment goals. Only rarely does the psychiatrist attempt to do psychotherapy with these patients. Yet, as the case presented below clearly demonstrates, even when the underlying organic defect cannot be corrected, and normal mental functioning restored, this does not rule out the possibility that these patients can be helped, by appropriate psychological techniques, to adjust to their deficits in mental and intellectual functioning.

> Mrs. G., a 68-year-old former actress, was admitted to the hospital with confusion and memory impairment so severe that she could not remember her name. Mrs. G. had a history of long-standing arteriosclerotic heart disease and hypertension, which had caused occasional dizziness, confusion, and memory lapses. But the realization that this time she had forgotten her own name had precipitated a panic.

An immediate psychiatric consultation was requested. The patient's staff doctor, who thought the patient was "about to jump out of her skin," was concerned that she might have a hypertensive crisis momentarily. In addition, the patient had a tachycardia that was related, in part, to her anxiety. Some members of the staff felt that this critically ill patient should be transferred to the psychiatric unit. But the general consensus was that Mrs. G. suffered from an irreversible organic syndrome, and that treatment should be limited to medication that would alleviate her anxiety.

The routine mental status examination administered at the outset by the psychiatrist confirmed that Mrs. G.'s mental functions were significantly impaired and that her reactive anxiety seemed to be further increasing her deficits in a vicious circle.

Later, when she had responded to anti-anxiety medication, the psychiatrist learned that Mrs. G. had begun to "go downhill" two years earlier when one of her daughters had died. It was evident that time had not softened this blow; Mrs. G. continued to mourn the loss of her daughter. The psychiatrist also learned that the period of confusion and disorientation that had necessitated Mrs. G.'s hospital admission had its onset at a time when she was experiencing a resurgence of the feelings of despair and helplessness associated with her daughter's death.

There was no doubt of the presence of an organic brain syndrome in this patient, and the use of anti-anxiety medication was clearly indicated. But in view of the acute onset of Mrs. G.'s mental symptoms, it was apparent that the patient also required a careful cardiovascular assessment, which, in fact, revealed digitalis toxicity. Thus, treatment tactics for two facets of Mrs. G.'s problem were clearly defined. Stelazine was used to treat her behavioral disturbance (anxiety, panic), and the acute mental concomitants of her organic dysfunction were alleviated by reducing her prescribed dosage of digitalis, and increasing her use of diuretics. It was then necessary to turn to Mrs. G.'s psychological dysfunction—her inability to cope with her environment.

It was important to allow Mrs. G. to complete the "work of mourning," and she was encouraged to ventilate her anger and hurt over the loss of her daughter. Inevitably, she had some feelings of guilt as well. This became apparent when she revealed her fantasy, which the psychiatrist was able to dispel, that she would die from phlebitis, as her daughter had. This led to a discussion of the anxiety she had experienced recently when she had had to have a toe amputated, her continuing anxiety about her failing health, and the disappointment she felt when she was forced to retire from the stage. In fact, although she could no longer use the theater as a vehicle for narcissistic gratification, as she talked it became apparent that Mrs. G. had retained many of the qualities that had made her a successful actress.

Despite the fact that she was beginning to recover from her acute organic syndrome, she still suffered significant organic impairment as a result of her chronic, irreversible syndrome. Yet she had not lost the capacity to relate to others. The ward staff was completely captivated by her wit and charm. Obviously, she was not a candidate for a wheelchair, nor was she meant to spend the rest of her life "off stage." She welcomed the psychiatrist's suggestion that she join a group for senior citizens, and serve as a consultant to a group of golden-agers who were planning to stage a play. Her response to the psychiatrist's supportive interventions was: "I can go on. I didn't know there was a place for me. Maybe my worries made me forget my name. It's like stage fright. I forgot my lines."

In contrast to Mrs. T., whose behavior was modified solely by treatment of her organic dysfunction, Mrs. G.'s behavioral disturbance was alleviated by treatment of both her organic and psychological dysfunctions.

Thus it becomes clear that the psychiatrist has the potential capacity to enhance the medical and psychological care of patients with organic brain syndromes and to enlist the cooperation and involvement of the internist in his efforts to this end. However, if he is to achieve this goal he must apply his knowledge of ego psychology; understand and be able to interpret the data derived from the mental status examination, and develop more refined techniques for the assessment of mental functioning in the medically ill; and, finally, he must extend his treatment goals beyond management of the acute symptoms of the organic brain syndromes.

REFERENCES

1. Schwartz F, Strain JJ: Personal communication, 1975
2. Engel G: Delirium. In Freedman AM, Kaplan HI (eds): The Comprehensive Textbook of Psychiatry. Baltimore, Williams & Wilkins, 1967, pp. 711–716
3. Simon A, Kahan RB: Acute brain syndromes in geriatric patients. Psych Res Reports 16:8, 1963
4. Freud S: Project for a scientific psychology. In Standard Edition of the Complete Psychological Works of Sigmund Freud, Vol. 1. London, Hogarth, 1966, pp. 283–387
5. Goldstein K: After-Effects of Brain Injuries in War. New York, Grune & Stratton, 1942
6. Talland GA: Deranged Memory: A Psychonomic Study of the Amnesic Syndrome. New York, Academic Press, 1965
7. Schwartz F: Personal communication
8. Mattis S: The mental status examination for organic mental syndrome in the elderly patient. In Bellak L, Karasu TB (eds): The Concise Handbook of Geriatric Psychiatry. New York, Grune & Stratton, in press
9. Mattis S: Personal communication
10. Shands H: An outline of the process of recovery from severe trauma. AMA Arch Neurol Psychiatry 13:403, 1955.

Part II
Specific Clinical Issues

Commentary

The clinical issues included in this section represent some of the most difficult problems encountered in medical practice, illustrate in concrete terms of deficits in current hospital care, and further explain the origins and consequences of these deficits.

All of these clinical issues have both a psychological and a physiological component, but they are usually approached conceptually and clinically from one vantage point or the other. To understand the origins of this "split," one must understand the evolution of medical and psychiatric research over the past fifty years. Advances in medicine have fostered concern with the body and a consequent undertreatment of the patient's psychological needs. In contrast, early psychiatric investigations of the relationship between psyche and soma resulted in an overemphasis on the psychological causes and cures of physical illness. As Edward Sachar points out in Chapter 5, these theories have not been validated by contemporary research criteria. In contrast to Sachar we feel the correlations between personality and various psychosomatic illnesses have theoretical and practical importance. They may offer clues for future research on psychophysiological relationships; certainly, they provide important insights into patients' psychological reactions to physical illness. Regardless of the etiology of their disease, these patients have somatopsychic reactions and/or reactions to their hospitalization which merit psychological evaluation and intervention, when indicated. Psychosomatic patients are frequently denied the benefits of this approach. In fact, even when such intervention is mandatory, these patients are rarely referred for psychiatric consultation.

Within the past twenty years the mind–body split has taken on a new character. There has been an intense preoccupation with the biological origins and management of psychological disorders, whether these occur in the medically ill or the psychiatrically ill, and as a consequence the dynamic psychological approach, which is an essential component of holistic patient care, has lost favor. The evaluation of the efficacy of the biological approach to endogenous depression advocated in Chapter 6 lies beyond the scope of the present discussion. However, even with these patients, we would question the value of any diagnostic assessment or treatment plan that is not based on consideration of the whole patient (that is, both biological and psychological considerations). Furthermore, in our view common psycho-dynamic issues—such as pathological reactions to loss—that course through depressive reactions and even grief in some cases are obscured by diagnostic formulations based primarily on descriptive symptomatology. The case described by Sachar of grief that ended in suicide might be understood by some as an example of a severe depressive illness secondary to multiple losses.

These clinical issues share certain features on a deeper level as well. They have not been precisely defined in terms of their origin, diagnosis, and management. Therefore, they automatically evoke certain stressful reactions in the physician—for example, feelings of impotence, guilt, bewilderment, uncertainty, and anger—all of which will affect his attitude toward, and management of, the patient. For example, he may abandon his patient emotionally or physically, or undertreat or overtreat the patient's physical or psychological problems. These reactions reach their apex in the doctor who must care for a patient who is dying and have crucial consequences for the patient's management. Although the stresses to which the dying patient is subject have been discussed at length in the literature, the stresses this clinical situation evokes in his doctor have not been adequately formulated. The discussion in Chapter 11 by Spikes and Holland constitutes a valuable contribution in this area.

Patients with hypochondriasis, patients in pain, and surgical patients may evoke the same stressful reactions in their doctors. For example, physicians frequently overtreat or undertreat such patients. The hypochondriacal patient is overdiagnosed, overtreated with medications (and balms), and overreassured that there is nothing wrong with his body. However, the psychological problem that lies at the root of the hypochondriasis is neglected. Since the internist is the primary caretaker of the hypochondriac, he must know how to handle the psychological aspects of this illness. The conceptualization of hypochondriasis in Chapter 7 can be further clarified by the newer metapsychological hypotheses about the self and of narcissism in particular, which address the seeming paradox that Altman presents: the patient withdraws from external objects but at the same time displays an intense desire for an external need gratifying object (often in the form of the doctor) who is admiring, tolerant, and undemanding of any recognition for himself. Although the psychological understanding of hypochondriasis is incomplete, we agree that a central issue of treatment is to provide a therapeutic (object) relationship that allows for the maintenance of the patient's emotional homeostasis without the promise of cure.

Pain is undertreated psychologically and pharmacologically. And last, but not least, it is generally recognized that surgical patients, who always need psychological care, both before and after their surgery, are the least likely to receive it. In Chapter 10, Baudry and Wiener concentrate on the neglect of the surgical patient's psychological needs by his doctor. But as other chapters in this book show, the factors to which they attribute the surgeon's failure to enlist appropriate psychiatric support occur in all fields of medicine. Furthermore, the special need of the surgical patient to view his surgeon as omnipotent ("the magic of the knife") and on a pedestal, in itself contributes to the distance between them.

The tendency to function at one extreme or another—to undertreat or overtreat—is reflected in the overuse or underuse of psychotropic drugs for the medically ill by internists and psychiatrists alike. For example, the minor tranquilizers are used excessively, and the major tranquilizers are not used often enough. Moreover, the range of drugs in the physician's armamentarium is not broad enough; his repertoire should, but often does not, include such drugs as antihistamines, paraldehyde, and phenobarbital. We advocate appropriate use of psychotropic drugs in appropriate dosage. However, we do not endorse the current tendency by some psychiatrists and internists to indiscriminately prescribe these drugs as the sole treatment approach to normal adaptive and maladaptive reactions to illness and hospitalization.

The issues discussed in this section merit more detailed elucidation. However, contributors were encouraged to limit "coverage" of their subject, in accordance with the stated purpose of this "primer." Thus the aim of these chapters is to alert the internist to the need to extend his armamentarium, and to alert the psychiatrist to those problem areas in which his skills and specialized knowledge are most needed.

Chapter 5*

The Current Status of Psychosomatic Medicine

Edward J. Sachar

What ever happened to "psychosomatic medicine"? For at least two decades after World War II, it was generally accepted in psychiatry and in popular culture that certain illnesses were "psychosomatic"—that is, psychological factors played a necessary and specific role in the predisposition, onset, or course of the disease. Everyone "knew," for example, that there was a peptic ulcer personality, a hypertensive personality, and so forth. Where did these ideas come from? How have they fared in the light of recent research? What does "psychosomatic medicine" mean today?

The man who really established psychosomatic concepts as part of psychiatric thought was Franz Alexander.[1] He and his colleagues made their original observations on a relatively small group of patients with a variety of medical illnesses who were in psychoanalysis and psychoanalytic therapy. Drawing on the work of earlier psychosomatic theorists and investigators, Alexander modified their concepts and synthesized a persuasive formulation of the psychological processes active in the illnesses he defined as psychosomatic. It is important to recognize that these formulations were not only psychoanalytic but also psychophysiological hypotheses.

According to Alexander, Flanders Dunbar[2] was correct in her notion of specific personality factors associated with particular illnesses, but what was specific was not the profile of superficial personality traits but rather a particular underlying, unresolved neurotic conflict. This conflict when it became intensified could exacerbate or precipitate the illness. The psychosomatic mechanism involved was not conversion, however, as Felix Deutsch[3] and his co-workers believed. Rather, the affective component of the conflict, denied external expression, was discharged excessively into internal visceral and vegetative pathways of the type described by Walter Cannon, and this chronic internal discharge resulted eventually in somatic

* An earlier version of this paper was published in *Psychiatric Annals,* 2:22–35, 1972.

disturbances and organic lesions. Alexander also considered some constitutional organ vulnerability to be a necessary, though not sufficient, cause of psychosomatic illness.

In one of his most influential formulations, Alexander reported that patients with peptic ulcer were revealed by psychoanalytic investigation to be in severe conflict about their oral dependent strivings, which were inconsistent with their ego ideals. These strivings, denied gratification and external expression, were discharged through the hypothalamus along autonomic pathways to the stomach, which behaved as if continually hungry for mother's milk, with excessive acid secretion and eventual ulceration. As another example, in ulcerative colitis, the disappointment in, resentment, and sense of loss of the depended-upon loved one could not be expressed; the patient responded by a desperate effort to please the loved one in the archaic way learned during toilet training—by producing bowel movement after bowel movement, leading to explosive diarrhea and eventual ulceration. Similar formulations were developed for rheumatoid arthritis, bronchial asthma, essential hypertension, Graves' disease, and neurodermatitis.

Alexander's hypotheses, which he felt were strongly supported by his psychoanalytic data, inspired a torrent of psychosomatic research. Most of it was concerned with confirming his psychoanalytic correlations rather than his psychophysiological ideas. The culmination of the correlational research has only recently been published in the volumes entitled *Psychosomatic Specificity,*[4] after long delays occasioned by efforts to cope with the complex control issues involved. The study indicates that a panel of analysts trained in Alexander's formulations could correctly match edited transcripts of psychiatric interviews with various types of psychosomatic patients to the correct medical diagnosis more than three times more frequently than chance—and, in fact, twice as successfully as a panel of internists. There were variations in the analysts' success rate from illness to illness, but their overall results were statistically significant.

Yet, despite the rigorous efforts to edit all medical clues from the interview transcripts, certain control problems gradually have been perceived as insurmountable in studying patients with well-established illnesses. A chronic illness seriously affecting an organ system and occupying a patient's concerns cannot help but have subtle yet pervasive somato-psychic effects, coloring perception and mental imagery with the psychological issues evoked by his symptoms. For example, what latent conflicts are likely to be stirred up by the need to deal with explosive, uncontrolled diarrhea or with constant hunger pangs and the need to keep drinking milk? Would not severe bronchial asthma in childhood be expected to shape personality development, as a consequence of the particular stresses and altered relationships imposed by the disease? Again, doesn't the patient who is continually and uneasily aware of his hypertensive potential also sense at some level that becoming angry will raise his blood pressure and possibly harm him? Such patients could be expected to develop inhibitions around expressions of hostility much like the coronary patient who said, "I am at the mercy of the first scoundrel who can make me angry!" Patients also develop fantasies about their illnesses and their causes; the analyst is misled if he takes the patient's after-the-fact symbolization of his illness for the psychic mechanism that caused it. As another example, many patients respond to illness and hospitalization with a sense of personal failure and helplessness, feelings that may color their retrospective description of the life events preceding the illness; it would be easy to mistake this psychic reaction for the emotional state that actually helped precipitate the illness.

We can hardly dismiss all the psychological correlates of psychosomatic conditions as psychic responses to illness; this is particularly difficult to do in the case of personality traits that as best as can be determined retrospectively, were prominent long before the illness broke out. Yet, it has been apparent for some time that correlative psychosomatic research would have to move to prospective studies. If it were only possible to find a biochemical or physiological marker to identify patients likely to develop the illnesses before they actually become manifest!

Arthur Mirsky was among the first to realize the advantage, indeed the necessity, of such an approach. Utilizing the fact that plasma pepsinogen levels roughly correlate with gastric secretion of acid and pepsin and that hypersecretors of acid are highly at risk for development of peptic ulcers, Weiner, Thaler, Reiser, and Mirsky[5] screened a large number of soldiers for plasma pepsinogen concentration, and so identified an asymptomatic hypersecreting group, as well as a hyposecreting group. Applying Alexander's formulations to psychological test data, it was possible to identify correctly 51 percent of the hyposecretors and 71 percent of the hypersecretors. Retrospective analysis of the psychological criteria permitted selection of characteristics more specifically associated with hypersecretion, but the study was never repeated on a new group of subjects, using the modified formulations.

In many ways, it is a pity that this significant prospective research in peptic ulcer has not been replicated or pursued. Other centers, however, have attempted to use a similar physiological marker technique for prospective psychosomatic studies. Wallerstein and his colleagues[6] applied Alexander's formulation for psychological predisposition to Graves' disease to women with areas of increased radioactive iodine uptake in the thyroid not as yet associated with any manifest clinical symptoms. They found that there was a tendency for women with these subclinical "hot spots" to be martyr-like people who from an unusually early stage in life had taken on heavy responsibilities, a finding that was consistent with the views of

Alexander, Ham, and their group.[4] In one randomly sampled group of normals, the ability of the investigators to select women with the thyroid abnormalities from controls was highly significant, although in other groups they were less successful. A subsequent longitudinal study[7] of a group of women with the hot spots indicated that the spots tended to wax and wane with the degree of nonspecific life strain with the implication that frank hyperthyroidism could well occur in the future.

These data raise some puzzling questions, however. Weiner[8] has pointed out that the type of hyperthyroidism likely to occur in women with hot spots is probably toxic nodular goiter, a very different illness in its endocrinology from the Graves' disease originally studied by Alexander's group. Furthermore, the waxing and waning of the hot spots in association with nonspecific life stress does not exactly support the specificity hypothesis, that is, that a specific neurotic conflict gives rise to a particular illness.

In other words, although it may be possible to demonstrate, even prospectively, that patients with certain personality constellations also happen to be more prone to certain illnesses, it is another assumption that a particular neurotic conflict exerts a specific influence on the clinical course of a disease. From another point of view, accepting that states of acute emotional distress can somehow increase the likelihood of illness in a vulnerable organ, and that different personalities become anxious in response to different stresses, is not the same as claiming that a particular neurosis perpetuates a specific illness. Indeed, it is this aspect of Alexander's theory dealing with pathogenesis that has fared the worst in contemporary research. If a specific area of neurotic conflict were really pathogenic in these disorders, it would be possible to demonstrate that resolution of the conflict through psychoanalysis or psychotherapy would alter the long-term clinical course of the disease. This has not really been demonstrated, however, in part because of the failure to do adequate medical follow-ups of psychotherapeutically treated psychosomatic patients and in part because our understanding of the natural history of the illnesses under study is still inadequate.

For example, there is still no good evidence (with adequate follow-up and adequate controls) that psychoanalysis favorably alters the ultimate course of peptic ulcer disease. Again, many analysts have claimed to have cured essential hypertension with analytic therapy. But nonmalignant essential hypertension, according to current concepts, is a disease that has at least two stages. First, there is a labile phase in which blood pressure may rise for days or weeks in association with dietary indiscretions, life stresses, and other undetermined factors, but following which the blood pressure typically normalizes in response to rest, sedation, diet, and other supportive measures designed to relieve stress. Many such patients, however, will eventually enter a second, fixed phase in which the diastolic pressure remains permanently elevated in the absence of specific antihypertensive agents. Thus it appears that many of the apparently positive analytic results have been temporary remissions obtained in the labile phase. There is no evidence as yet from long-term follow-up that such analyzed patients are less likely than controls to have subsequent exacerbations of hypertension or are less likely to enter the fixed stage of the disease with fixed elevation of blood pressure.

As another example, ulcerative colitis can take several forms, each with a different course and prognosis. One form has been recently recognized to be a separate illness altogether, Crohn's disease of the colon. Another type is, from the beginning, exclusively restricted to the proctosigmoid colon and runs a relatively benign course, compared to the diffuse disseminated form. Even such a careful follow-up study of psychotherapeutically treated ulcerative colitis patients as that conducted by Karush, Daniels, O'Connor, and their associates[9] failed to distinguish adequately the medical types of ulcerative colitis under study or to include a control group of colitis patients treated without psychotherapy; and so it is hard to determine whether psychotherapy does have an enduring effect on the course of the disease in its various forms.

The more that is understood of the pathophysiology of the psychosomatic illnesses, the less tenable seem Alexander's psychophysiological formulations. He spoke, for example, of the hostility of the rheumatoid arthritis patient producing increased tension in the joint muscles, leading to arthritic lesions. We know now, however, that the muscle tension is secondary to the painful inflammation and that the primary lesion is certainly elsewhere, possibly in the cells of the synovial membrane. Alexander's psychophysiological formulation of ulcerative colitis was similarly based on a misconception. Engel[10] was the first to point out that Alexander assumed severe diarrhea to be the cardinal symptom in ulcerative colitis, with ulcerations of the mucosa occurring as a result; in fact, the initial observable lesion is a change in the mucosa associated with bleeding, and diarrhea is a secondary manifestation. If Alexander's formulations were correct, one would expect patients with the spastic colon–irritable bowel syndrome to go on to develop ulcerative colitis, which they do not. Indeed, a viral etiology of both Crohn's disease and ulcerative colitis is now suspected. As yet another example, the role of sympathetic tone in essential hypertension, critical to Alexander's formulation, is now seen as only one element in an extremely complex pathophysiological system to which significant contributions are made by hormonal factors such as renin, angiotensin, aldosterone, and so forth.

In summary, then, none of the classical psychosomatic theories of Alexander, particularly as they apply to the diseases he emphasized, has received strong support by modern research. On the other hand, another disease, not included by Alexander in his psychosomatic group, has in recent years been the subject of considerable psychosomatic interest: a series of prospective studies of healthy men, initiated by Friedman and Rosenman[11] and others, have suggested that subjects with a particular personality constellation are more prone to develop coronary artery disease in later life. These prospective investigations were a part of several long-range, multifactorial studies of coronary artery disease launched in the late 1940s and 1950s. The personality profile, termed the "Type A" constellation, includes such surface features as upward strivings; a sense of urgency about, and excessive consciousness of, deadlines; a driven quality of speech; and a tendency to be impatient. It is obviously an exceedingly difficult task to match groups for such significant intervening variables as cigarette smoking, diet, exercise habits, obesity, and so forth, but thus far the results seem to be holding up.

With this one exception, the focus of interest in psychosomatic illness has shifted from specific to nonspecific psychological factors. Indeed, research begun by Rahe, Følstad, Bergan, and their co-workers,[12] and subsequently pursued by other investigators, has produced an impressive body of evidence that life stresses and life changes of all types substantially increase the likelihood of falling ill from virtually any disease! In the usual investigation of this type, subjects fill out a life events inventory, in which anything from change of a job to death of a spouse can be checked off. Each item is assigned a score, derived previously from surveys of people's opinions as to the emotional significance of such events. Again and again, it appears that subjects with high scores become ill during the next six months with everything from heart attacks to cancer to influenza with greater frequency than low-scoring subjects.

But what are the physiological mechanisms by which life stress, specific or nonspecific, leads to somatic disease? This question has emerged as the central problem in psychosomatic research of the past twenty years. The strategy of these recent studies varies radically from that of the past, however, with the appreciation of the enormous complexity of the illnesses previously considered psychosomatic. Diseases like peptic ulcer, ulcerative colitis, neurodermatitis, and rheumatoid arthritis are seen as psychosomatically unresearchable at this time, because medical research has not yet determined the nature of the primary disorders. How can one study the pathways by which emotional states lead to flare-ups of rheumatoid arthritis, if one does not know what system is basically awry in that illness? Is rheumatoid arthritis an autoimmune disease, a latent viral infection, an enzymatic defect of the synovial membrane cells, or a collagen disease? The strategies of psychosomatic research would be quite different in each instance. If one wanted to measure the relevant somatic response in the arthritic to a given psychological stimulus, one would hardly know whether to take a blood sample, a muscle biopsy, or a sample of synovial fluid.

What has happened is that many psychosomatic researchers have for the time being shifted their attention away from complex disease entities and focused instead on studying psychological influences on somatic systems whose responses can be measured, systems that may eventually prove to be implicated in somatic illnesses of many types, not just in those designated by Alexander and his co-workers. The scope of this research has become quite large. A few examples will be described here to illustrate some of these new directions.

In Alexander's time, the major recognized psychophysiological pathway was that of the autonomic nervous system. Miller[13] recently extended the studies of autonomic responsivity to paradigms of instrumental conditioning. Their initial results suggested that it was possible to "learn" autonomic response patterns, with the corollary that animals and people could be "trained" to raise and lower blood pressure, alter vascular flow, change pulmonary resistance, and so forth. It has not been possible to replicate these original exciting observations, however. Nevertheless, the biofeedback experiments stimulated by this research continue, and may yet prove to have therapeutic possibilities.

Since the 1950s, another major psychosomatic system has been identified and studied—the neuroendocrine apparatus. We have learned in the past twenty years that hypothalamic centers regulate the secretion of virtually all the hormones of the anterior pituitary,[14] and it has also become clear that psychological stimuli can have important influences on these neuroendocrine control mechanisms.[15] Among the hormones that have been shown to be highly sensitive to psychological stress in both animals and man are ACTH, cortisol, growth hormone, prolactin, testosterone, and perhaps TSH and thyroxine. Because this group of hormones from the pituitary and its target glands affect virtually every biochemical process in the body, it is obvious that the neuroendocrine system could play a significant role in somatic disease.

Related to these areas of psychoendocrine and psychophysiological investigation are the burgeoning studies in development psychophysiology. Some of this research has as its premise that just as there appear to be critical periods in development when psychological patterns can be imprinted, there also may be critical periods for the imprinting of physiological response patterns. Several investigators[16, 17] are exploring the possibility that early experiences in the rat can affect the nature of its subsequent adrenocortical responses to stress. Hofer and Weiner[18] are investigating the role of early maternal separation in the subsequent balance of parasympathetic and sympathetic tone in regulating the heart. In the human neonate, developmental psychophysiological research has focused on identifying some of the inborn constitutional differences between infants in psychophysiological reactivity,[19, 20] traits that may someday help account for the differences between people in their susceptibility to certain illnesses.

In the areas of cardiovascular physiology, Henry and his colleagues[21] have conducted a series of ingenious experiments demonstrating that altering the psychosocial environment of mice has dramatic and enduring effects on their blood pressure. With increasing crowding, social disorganization, and confrontations over dominance, the mice develop hypertension with pathological consequences—experimental observations that might make the urban dweller uncomfortable indeed.

Psychological influences on the gastrointestional system have been studied systematically by Weiss.[22] By altering the nature of the conditioned psychological stress and the range of coping devices available to the animal under observation, Weiss has been able to strikingly increase and decrease the amount of gastric ulceration produced.

Yet another field of investigation that has potential for clarifying psychosomatic mechanisms is the study of sleep physiology. The stage of dreaming or rapid eye movement (REM) sleep is associated with profound psychophysiological activation of many systems. Of particular interest for the psychosomaticist are the findings of Kales and Tau[23] that the peptic ulcer patient secretes the bulk of his nighttime acid during the REM periods, and the observations by Nowtin and his associates[24] that patients with nocturnal angina episodes experience them almost exclusively during REM periods.

Although I have touched only briefly on a few of the new areas of psychosomatic research, it can be seen that the field appears to have moved far from what had been traditionally regarded as the sphere of psychosomatic medicine. These studies are making major contributions to our understanding of psychosomatic processes, both normal and abnormal. There is every reason to believe that with increased medical understanding of the pathogenesis of diseases such as atherosclerosis and rheumatoid arthritis, a linkage will eventually be made between the two growing spheres of research. When and if this occurs, we can look forward to the development of a true science of psychosomatic medicine. In the interim, the liaison psychiatrist will wisely refrain from excessive psychologizing in his approach to patients with peptic ulcer or rheumatoid arthritis, but he will be more aware than ever of the vulnerability of every patient's physiology to the stresses and strains of everyday life.

REFERENCES

1. Alexander F: Psychosomatic Medicine. New York, Norton, 1950
2. Dunbar F: Emotions and Bodily Changes. New York, Columbia Univ Press, 1954
3. Deutsch F (ed): On the Mysterious Leap from the Mind to the Body: A Workshop Study on the Theory of Conversion. New York, International Universities Press, 1959
4. Alexander F, French T (eds): Psychosomatic Specificity, Vol I. Chicago, Univ Chicago Press, 1968
5. Weiner H, Thaler M, Reiser M, Mirsky A: Etiology of duodenal ulcer. 1: Relation of specific psychological characteristics to rate of gastric secretion (serum pepsinogen). Psychosom Med 19:1, 1957
6. Wallerstein RS, Holzman TS, Voth HM, Uhr N: Thyroid "hot spots," a psychophysiological study. Psychosom Med 27:508, 1965
7. Voth HM, Holzman TS, Katz JB, Wallerstein RS: Thyroid "hot spots": their relationship to life stress. Psychosom Med 32:561, 1970
8. Weiner H: The specificity hypothesis revisited. Psychosom Med 32:543, 1970
9. Karush A, Daniels G, O'Connor J, et al: Response to psychotherapy in chronic ulcerative colitis. I. Psychosom Med 30:255, 1968; II. Psychosom Med 31:201, 1969
10. Engel G: Studies of ulcerative colitis. II: The nature of the somatic process and the adequacy of psychosomatic hypotheses. Am J Med 16: 416, 1954
11. Friedman M, Rosenman RH: Type A behavior pattern: its association with coronary heart disease. Ann Clin Res 3:300–312, 1971
12. Rahe RH, Følstad I, Bergan T, et al: A model for life changes and illness research. Arch Gen Psychiatry 31:172–177, 1974
13. Miller NE: Learning of visceral and glandular responses. Science 163:434, 1969
14. Martini L, Ganong WF (eds): Neuroendocrinology. New York, Academic Press, 1966
15. Mason J: Organization of neuroendocrine mechanisms. Psychosom Med 30:565–808, 1968
16. Ader R: Adrenocortical function and the measurement of "emotionality." Ann NY Acad Sci 159:791–805, 1969
17. Levine S: The pituitary-adrenal system and the developing brain. In DeWeid D, Weijnen J (eds): Progress in Brain Research, Vol 32. Pituitary, Adrenal and the Brain. New York, Elsevier, 1970
18. Hofer MA, Weiner H: Development of mechanisms of cardiorespiratory responses to maternal deprivation in rat pups. Psychosom Med 33:353, 1971
19. Bridger W, Birns B, Blank M: A comparison of behavioral ratings and heart rate measurements in human neonates. Psychosom Med 27:123, 1965
20. Lipton EL, Steinschneider A, Richmond JB: Autonomic function in the neonate. VII: Maturational changes in cardiac control. Child Dev 37:1, 1966
21. Henry JP, Meehan JP, Stephens P: The use of psychosocial stimulation to

induce prolonged systolic hypertension in mice. Psychosom Med 29:408–432, 1967

22. Weiss JM: Influences of psychological variables on stress-induced pathology. Physiological Emotions and Psychosomatic Illness. CIBA Foundation Symposium 8 (new series) Excerpta Medica, Amsterdam, 1972

23. Kales A, Tau T: Sleep alterations and medical illness. In Kales A (ed): Sleep Physiology and Pathology. Philadelphia, Lippincott, 1969, p. 148

24. Nowlin JB, Troyer, WG, Jr, Collins WS, et al: Association of nocturnal angina pectoris with dreaming. Ann Intern Med 63:1040, 1965

Chapter 6

Evaluating Depression in the Medical Patient

Edward J. Sachar

Depressive experiences are ubiquitous among the medically ill, yet the proper evaluation and treatment of the depressed medical patient remains one of the most difficult tasks for the internist and psychiatrist. In part, this is because the term "depression" is a broad and ambiguous one, encompassing several different conditions, each with a differing etiology and with a different treatment of choice. Distinguishing among these conditions is not easy, since their clinical phenomena overlap, and many patients present mixed pictures. Another complicating factor is medical illness itself, which can produce many symptoms, such as fatigue and anorexia, that ordinarily are used in the differential diagnosis of depressive disorders.

In this brief discussion I will focus on five conditions associated with depressive symptoms: true depressive illnesses of the unipolar or bipolar (manic-depressive) type, grief and loss reactions, neurotic characterological depressions, primary medical conditions that frequently produce depressive symptomatology, and drug-induced depressions.

DEPRESSIVE ILLNESS

Although the clinical phenomena of depressive illnesses are well known to all psychiatrists and to most physicians, it will be useful for our discussion to review these disorders concisely, in the light of current thinking.

Typically the patient experiences symptoms that can be grouped roughly into "psychological" and "somatic" categories. Among the most common psychological symptoms are depressed mood; a profound, pervasive loss of interest and pleasure; feelings of worthlessness; pessimism; indecisiveness; ruminative worries; and a loss of emotional responsivity to the environment. Additional frequent symptoms are pervasive anxiety, suicidal thoughts, and guilty self-recriminations. It is part of the definition of depressive illness, and a major distinction from grief reactions, that these psychological concerns are out of proportion to whatever realistic problems confront the patient, and that they may reach delusional intensity. Attempts to correct the patient's unrealistic ideas are unsuccessful. It is also important to note that, in contrast to grief reactions, feelings of sorrow are not common in depressive illness, although they may occur. Indeed, if asked, the typical patient will insist that the feeling he is experiencing is different from the feelings of grief he experienced in the past when he lost loved ones.

The most common somatic, or "vegetative" symptoms, are insomnia, particularly during the middle and end of the night; anorexia, sometimes leading to substantial weight loss; fatigue; psychomotor retardation or agitation; decreased libido; loss of aggressive drive, somatic pains, such as headaches, backaches, and toothaches; autonomic disturbances, such as constipation and dry mouth; and, sometimes, a diurnal variation in symptomatology, with the worst period in the morning.

These somatic symptoms have never been explained by a psychological theory, and they strongly suggest a disorder of hypothalamic function. It is important to recognize that depressive illness frequently presents primarily with the somatic symptoms, while the psychological symptoms may be relatively slight. European psychiatrists have called such syndromes "vital" depressions, while the American school has sometimes labeled these cases "denied" or "masked" depressions. It now appears that these latter terms are misnomers in that they imply the patient is covering up his "true" depressed feelings. Again, psychiatrists have sometimes construed the pains and other somatic symptoms of the illness as conversion reactions; they are not. In fact, depressive illness is as much a somatic condition as a psychological one, and some cases merely present with more symptoms of the one than of the other. When this happens, the internist can easily be misled, and pursue to an inappropriate degree an organic work-up and medical treatment:

> For more than a year, Mr. P., a 60-year-old piano teacher, had complained to his dentist of ill-fitting dentures, to his chiropodist of pains in his feet, and to his general practitioner of fatigue. The dentist had refitted his dentures several times, the chiropodist had tried several procedures, and the general practitioner had been giving him Vitamin B-12 injections, all to no avail. His wife finally called the physician to say she had discovered her husband on the roof, contemplating jumping to his death. He was promptly admitted to a psychiatric ward.
>
> Mr. P. was found to be an agreeable, well-dressed man, who was able to smile appropriately during the interview. He acknowledged

feeling depressed, but only about his somatic problems, which he said, were a "life and death" matter to him. A careful review of his functioning revealed, however, that he had no appetite and had lost ten pounds in the last three months; that he regularly awakened at 4 A.M., and then ruminated constantly about his teeth and feet; that he had lost his previous keen interests in reading and music, and had even allowed his beloved piano to go untuned; that nothing gave him pleasure; and that this usually meticulous man had lost the energy and will to do things that he knew were important. "I tell myself I'll do it tomorrow, but tomorrow never comes." The psychiatrist also learned that Mr. P. had had a serious depression five years previously, which, like this one, had had no obvious precipitant. The patient made a dramatic recovery after six electro-convulsive treatments, returned to full functioning, and subsequently saw his teeth and feet problems as minor annoyances, easily coped with.

This example illustrates some features of the strategy of differentially diagnosing a depressive illness from a primary medical illness: taking a thorough inventory of possible depressive symptoms will usually reveal the characteristic syndrome of depressive illness. This syndrome is often termed "endogenous" depression, but this too is a misnomer, in that it suggests that there is never a psychological precipitant. Research involving careful anamneses has revealed that 35 to 40 percent of such patients have experienced significant psychological precipitants.[1] Of course, this is still substantially less than what is seen in grief reactions, where precipitants are universally present, and, in contrast to the grieving patient, the depressively ill patient is usually not affectively preoccupied with a loss or a disappointment. The key point, however, is that the precipitant of a depressive illness triggers off a syndrome that, in Gillespie's phrase[2] becomes relatively "autonomous" of the psychosocial environment. Klein[3] has termed these depressions "endogenomorphic," to emphasize the symptom picture, rather than the cause, and he underscores the pervasive loss of interests, pleasure, and emotional responsivity as cardinal diagnostic features.

Two additional historical characteristics of these depressions can aid in diagnosis. First, they are recurrent illnesses. Thus, Mr. P. had had a previous depressive episode, and five years after the one described, he had another. Angst,[4] in his careful longitudinal study of several hundred patients, calculated that 95 percent of patients experiencing an episode of severe depressive illness would have one or more subsequent attacks within ten years, and that in twenty years the average number of episodes is five for patients with unipolar illness (depressions only), and nine for patients with bipolar (manic-depressive) illness. This means that a previous episode of serious depression or mania substantially increases the likelihood that the present syndrome is another episode of the same illness (although patients with depressive diatheses certainly may experience normal grief reactions in intervals between episodes of illness).

Another important feature of depressive illness is that it runs in families (probably indicating significant genetic factors). About 15 to 20 percent of first degree relatives of patients with recurrent unipolar or bipolar depressive illness have histories of similar illness, which is at least ten times the incidence in the normal population.[5] Therefore, a family history of affective disorder also increases the likelihood that one is dealing with a depressive illness in the patient.

It is also important to be aware of certain physiological concomitants of depression that may create problems in the differential diagnosis of depression from medical illness. Many elderly patients with depressive illness manifest typical signs of a mild organic mental syndrome, with defects in memory, abstraction, and calculation; after recovery from the depression, the organic mental syndrome may markedly improve or completely clear.[6] The basis for this is unknown, although the hypothesized functional depletion in brain biogenic amine activity in depressive illness may play a role.[7] Again, these are endocrine disturbances associated with depression, which may confuse a work-up for endocrinopathy: many depressed patients markedly hypersecrete cortisol and hyposecrete growth hormone.[7] The reason for this is also unknown, although it may be another aspect of the apparent hypothalamic dysfunction seen in depressive illness. There are other possible biological markers of depressed patients, such as decreased urinary excretion of the noradrenalin metabolite MHPG, but none are sufficiently established as yet to serve as diagnostic aids.[7]

The episodes of illness in the great majority of cases are self-limited, with the course running about six to twelve months, if untreated. This means that the doctrinaire psychotherapist who is determined that such patients should "work through" their psychological conflicts unencumbered by antidepressant medication can be assured of a high success rate within six to twelve months of the onset of the syndrome. In fact, psychotherapy has no advantage over placebo, while proper antidepressant or electroconvulsive therapy (ECT) will be dramatically effective within four weeks in 80 to 90 percent of cases.[8] In other words, this is no longer an issue of the theoretical orientation or preference of the psychiatrist; rather, it is a matter of very poor practice if appropriate somatic therapy is not promptly instituted. Klein feels that the role of the psychotherapist in these cases is to help the patient accept somatic treatment. (The strategy of administering antidepressants to patients with medical complications is discussed in Chapter 9.) On the other hand, it should also be emphasized that there is no evidence that antidepressant medication is of any value in grief reactions, neurotic depressions, or "medical" depressions.[8]

Once the patient has recovered, a decision must also be made as to whether prophylactic medication should be instituted. Lithium prophylaxis has been shown in numerous studies to be remarkably effective in patients with either recurrent unipolar or bipolar depressive illness.[9, 10] The long-term morbidity of such patients is generally reduced to 20 percent of control groups. Certainly a patient who has had two or three serious episodes within five years should be begun on lithium, unless there are significant medical contraindications, and, in my view, failure to do so also is poor practice.

Supportive psychotherapy has an important role in helping these patients adjust to living with a chronic, relapsing illness, especially if maintenance drug therapy merely attenuates rather than eliminates the affective episodes. While insight-oriented psychotherapy has no proven value in preventing or treating the episodes, it may be indicated for other neurotic or character-ological problems the patient has.

GRIEF REACTIONS

Grief reactions are, of course, by far the most common depressive experiences of the medical patient. The range of losses facing the coronary patient, for example, is very large, and has been described in detail in Chapters 3 and 12. Here we may briefly review some of them: separation from his loved ones for many weeks of hospitalization; loss of ability to work; fear of loss of functions and of an independent way of life; fear of losing the esteem of family and colleagues who perceive him as an impaired or vulnerable person; a striking change in self-image; and, of course, fear of the loss of life itself. The neurological patient may have lost the power to walk, to speak, or to control bladder and bowel. Even less serious illnesses may alter one's self-image in terms of health, invulnerability, and physical attractiveness. It is no wonder that many patients become sad and despondent.

In differentiating these responses from depressive illness, it is worth keeping in mind that the mental preoccupations of melancholic patients are significantly out of proportion to the reality situation, while the grief responses are appropriate, and in a sense understandable. In order to make this distinction, however, the physician or consulting psychiatrist must learn from the patient what he is, in fact, responding to emotionally. This cannot be accomplished by a physician who has a stereotyped view of what patients ought to be able to tolerate or shrug off, or who overestimates what his hearty reassurance that "everything will be fine" actually accomplishes. The patient who, despite such a pep talk, remains upset may then be promptly given an antidepressant—usually in homeopathic doses, or, even more irrationally, on an as needed basis. Such failures in patient–doctor understanding and communication may at times be quite gross:

> When I was a psychiatric resident, I was called by the Chief Surgical Resident to see an Indian man with a severe leg burn, who had been tearful, despondent, and demanding insistently to see the doctors. It was the last behavior that had prompted the consultation request. The Chief Resident met me and handed me a paper with tightly written script. "Look at this. Is this the letter of a rational man?" I studied the letter briefly, and asked if he had read it. "I don't have to read it, the guy is a nut." The letter began, "Dear Dr. G., Forgive me for writing, but I am desperate. I have been here ten days, and no doctor has yet spoken with me to explain to me what will happen to my leg."

At times, however, the issue troubling the patient involves fantasy and unconscious elements that require careful exploration and unraveling by a psychiatrist:

> Mrs. B., a 37-year-old Catholic, married woman with diabetes, was admitted for reevaluation of her diabetic status, following complaints of persistent fatigue. She was observed by her physician to appear sad, to cry easily, and to express discouragement about her medical condition. He was unable to reassure her, and called a psychiatrist. The psychiatrist found her to be emotionally responsive, and eager to talk about her feelings. She acknowledged feeling blue and worried, but not to the point of losing interest in her family, and she was still able to enjoy things, although not as much as she had in the past. It was learned that she was thinking about an aunt who had had severe diabetic complications, including gangrenous toes and eventual blindness, and the patient feared she would suffer the same fate. When asked if she thought the illness was in any way a punishment, this religious woman replied, "Yes." She had begun to think so several months earlier when she had developed a severe vaginal monilial infection that had been resistant to treatment. At age 18, she had become pregnant out of wedlock by her present husband, and, although she immediately married, with the blessing of the priest and her family, she had always expected the sin to be punished. An intractable infection in the very place where she had sinned, making intercourse painful, seemed to be God's judgment at last. What had made her think her pregnancy such a sin was still unconscious, however. Her father, once idealized by her, had become a disgraced alcoholic, and, as a teenager, she had assumed her mother was continuing to be married to him in name only. To her surprise, her mother suddenly became pregnant, and the patient promptly became pregnant by her fiancé. The real

sin was the reevoked oedipal wish she had acted out at age 18.

The psychiatrist gave the patient the opportunity to talk about her feelings at the time of her pregnancy, and to see that there was a connection between her mother's pregnancy and her own. Discussing with her, in a tactful way, a little girl's warm feelings for her father was most helpful to her, as was an explanation of why it was so difficult to treat moniliasis in a diabetic. Her feelings of depression lifted in six sessions over a two-week period.

We may note from this example several features that distinguish Mrs. B.'s depression from depressive illness. While some issues were unconscious, the patient knew what we worrying her: her medical condition. And once the full meaning to her of her illness was understood, her emotional response seemed appropriate. Although she was worried, she did not ruminate constantly. She had not lost the ability to enjoy things, to respond affectively to her environment, and she retained her interest in her loved ones. Finally, she responded rapidly to psychotherapeutic intervention.

Grief reactions, of course, can also be overwhelming, as in the acutely bereaved, and may even lead to suicidal thoughts and actions:

> A 60-year-old dentist became deaf. A thorough work-up in the hospital revealed an inoperable brain tumor. Because he was a member of the medical profession, his doctors assumed he should be told the full facts of his fatal condition, including the possibility of blindness. Unfortunately, he was overwhelmed by the information and became deeply despondent, a state made worse by the sudden social isolation produced by his deafness. A further complication was the fact that his own doctor was away, and he was being treated by a substitute. When interviewed by the psychiatrist, he acknowledged, weeping, that he feared going blind more than death itself. Both deaf and blind, he would be totally dependent and would not even know whether anyone was in the room with him. He couldn't bear that—and contemplated committing suicide while he was still able to find his way about. When he was encouraged to feel that continued chemotherapy could arrest the tumor's progress, he felt he could go on, although he remained profoundly despondent. However, after his own doctor returned, the chemotherapy was judged to be ineffective and was halted, and he was discharged. Three days later, the patient jumped from a window, and ended his life.

Could antidepressants have been helpful to this man? We have no way of knowing, but we doubt it. It might have been more helpful to enlist his doctor and his family in a concerted effort to sustain his hope and allay his fears of abandonment, even if it meant continuing somatically ineffective chemotherapy.

NEUROTIC CHARACTEROLOGICAL DEPRESSIONS

"Neurotic depression" is a highly ambiguous term, used in many ways by different writers. I do not consider the previously described depressive reactions to loss "neurotic" depressions, although neurotic components were certainly apparent in each of them. The syndrome I have in mind might better be called depressive neurosis, or in Schildkraut's phrase,[11] chronic characterological depressions, emphasizing that these patients have lifelong significant character problems, which are often intensified by stress, including the stress of medical illness.

> Mrs. T., a 60-year-old, chronically unhappy, masochistic character, when hospitalized for treatment of mild congestive heart failure, dealt with her particular anxieties in the only way she knew—the same way that had previously alienated most of her family. She incessantly demanded constant attention from the staff, complaining bitterly at the same time that none of them really cared about her. "My doctor—such a big, famous man—is too busy to see me. He comes in the room and is gone before I can ask him anything." Filled with self-pity, she cried about her predicament, at the same time making it clear that no one appreciated how much she suffered. Any type of reassurance was met with remarks like, "It's easy for you to say, you're not sick!" and other guilt-engendering comments. Before long, nobody could tolerate her, and she had produced the very situation of isolation and resentment from the staff that she had feared.

In most cases of this type, the best the liaison psychiatrist can do is to support the staff, helping them understand that the patient's behavior is an entrenched part of her neurotic character, not to be taken personally. To protect the staff, the psychiatrist himself may need to act as a lightning rod for the patient's complaints, commiserating with her about her predicament, taking care to make his appointments regular, reliable, and of a consistent length. Antidepressants have been shown to be no more effective than placebo in such cases,[8] and their side effects may become a further focus for complaints. Sometimes a minor tranquilizer may diminish the patient's anxiety sufficiently to lessen the intensity of her pathological coping mechanisms. Unfortunately, while the staff (including the psychiatrist) may be privately praying for the patient's speedy recovery and prompt discharge, patients like Mrs. T., are prone to develop secondary gain from being in the hospital, and physical complaints may redouble as discharge approaches. The message is, "How can you throw a poor, sick woman like me out into the cold?" This may appear paradoxical, since until then the hospital had been described vividly by the patient as a virtual torture chamber. One recalls the cry of the woman at the Catskill mountain resort: "The food here is poison, poison, absolute poison! And such small portions!"

MEDICAL DEPRESSIONS

Certain primarily medical conditions frequently produce mental changes resembling primary depressive illness. Of course, many debilitating diseases produce lassitude, fatigue, discouragement, and so forth, but the illnesses listed below appear to be associated with more specific depressive phenomena. Indeed, frequently the first sign of the illness is a depressive syndrome. In none of these conditions are antidepressants of any proven value; only diagnosis and correction of the underlying medical illness will reverse the depression. The precise mechanisms by which depression is produced in these conditions is not known; very possibly elucidation of the pathophysiology of these medical depressions could provide clues to the psychobiology of endogenous depressive illness.

Endocrinopathies

Endocrine disorders and hormone therapy are associated with a variety of psychological disturbances, some of which closely mimic depressive disorders.[12] *Hyperparathyroidism* frequently produces a mental syndrome of fatigue, depressive mood, anhedonia, decreased self-esteem, pessimism, and inability to concentrate. The mental phenomena are directly related to the serum calcium concentration, particularly at levels of 11 to 14 mg. The syndrome can be immediately reversed by renal dialysis. In about one-third of the cases, *Cushing's syndrome* is associated with significant depression, which may be severe enough to involve suicidal thoughts and depressive delusions. Corticosteroid therapy can also produce similar depressive phenomena, but, in contrast to Cushing's syndrome, elation is more common than depression. *Hypothyroidism* is also typically associated with depressed mood, pessimism, and poor self-esteem, which is intensified by the organic mental syndrome produced by myxedema. *Premenstrual tension* is a syndrome that, in many women, is associated with depressed mood, pessimism, crying spells, and self-deprecation. Similar phenomena can be produced by oral contraceptives. While both estrogens and progesterone have been implicated in this disorder, it is still unclear what role these hormones play.

Viral Illnesses

Following a bout of influenza, many patients experience a period of asthenia that may last as long as four to six weeks after all objective signs of illness have disappeared. In an unpublished study conducted with Selwin Juter,[13] we found that after one influenza outbreak, about 25 percent of the patients in our sample reported depressed mood, pessimism, self-deprecation, diminished libido, anorexia, sleep disturbance, and decreased ambition three weeks after the illness had subsided. The causes of the asthenia are unknown. Infectious mononucleosis and infectious hepatitis frequently present with a syndrome of asthenia, anorexia, depressed mood, pessimism, and decreased ambition, and not infrequently the patients come first to a psychiatrist.

While the asthenia seen in these viral and postviral states is certainly linked somehow to sequelae of the original infection, the basis of the psychological depression is unclear. It may represent a secondary psychological reaction to feeling weak and tired. On the other hand, the association of the asthenic syndrome (which resembles the asthenia seen in endogenomorphic depression) and the depressive mental symptoms may be more fundamental, both perhaps reflecting a virally induced neurochemical change.

Occult Abdominal Neoplasms

A curious depressive syndrome has been observed in patients who are subsequently discovered to have carcinoma of the pancreas, stomach, or other abdominal organs. Such patients report fatigue, loss of normal ambitions and interests, depressed mood, and premonitions of doom. The symptoms occur at a time when the tumors are otherwise silent. Originally, it was thought that these depressive phenomena were specifically associated with pancreatic neoplasms, but it appears that they occur with other abdominal tumors, too.[14] The mechanism of the depressions is completely obscure; possibly through an as yet unknown somatosensory system, the patient receives preconscious signals of serious disease.

DRUG-INDUCED DEPRESSIONS

A careful review of the drug history should be a routine part of the evaluation of every depressed patient, since there are several medications that can provoke depressive reactions. We have already mentioned corticosteroids and oral contraceptives.

The most striking, clear-cut instance of a drug-induced depressive syndrome is that produced by reserpine. Initially, it was reported that as many as 15 percent of patients receiving the drug for hypertension experienced significant depressive phenomena, and it has subsequently become clear that among these depressive responses are a substantial number of true depressive illnesses.[15] The true depressive illnesses appear to be much more common among patients with previous histories of episodes of depressive illness. Often, removal of the drug in these cases is not sufficient to induce remission, and a course of antidepressant therapy is required. (These observations of the reserpine-induced depressions prompted the initial research that led to the catecholamine and idoleamine hypotheses of affective disorders.) In checking a patient's history for reserpine therapy, it is important to keep in mind that reserpine is incorporated as one of several ingredients in a number of combination drugs used for hypertension that have different brand names; sometimes neither the patient nor his physician is aware of this.

Alphamethyldopa (Aldomet), also used in the treatment of hypertension, can also provoke mild depressive phenomena, although it is not clear whether full-blown depressive illnesses can ensue.

Other drugs, particularly minor tranquilizers such as diazepam (Valium), may also exert a mild depressive effect on certain patients. Drug removal is sufficient to reverse the picture. Mild to severe transient depressive states also are common after withdrawal of amphetamines and other stimulant drugs. This poststimulant depression, sometimes called a crash, will generally pass, with supportive therapy, within a week.

In summary, I have described five classes of depressive syndromes, each with a different etiology and each calling for a different approach to treatment. Hopefully, the modern internist and psychiatrist will appreciate that as with describing a patient as "febrile," describing a patient as "depressed" is only the first step in what should be a rigorous, scientific evaluation.

REFERENCES

1. Paykel E, Myers J, Drenelt M, Klerman G: Life events and depression. Arch Gen Psychiatry 21:753–760, 1969
2. Gillespie RD: Clinical differentiation of types of depression. Guy's Hosp Reports 79:306–344, 1929
3. Klein DF: Endogenomorphic depression. Arch Gen Psychiatry 31:447–454, 1974
4. Angst J: Presentation to Denghausen Conference on Psychobiology of Depression. Aruba, March 1974

5. Perris C: Genetics of affective disorders. In Mendels J (ed): Biological Psychiatry. New York, Wiley, 1973, pp. 385–416
6. Kiloh LG: Pseudo-dementia. ACTA Psychiatr Scand 37:336, 1961
7. Sachar E, Coppen A: Biological aspects of affective psychoses. In Gaull G (ed): Biology of Brain Dysfunction. New York, Plenum, in press
8. Klein D, Davis J: Diagnosis and Drug Treatment of Psychiatric Disorders. Baltimore, Williams & Wilkins, 1969
9. Angst J, Weis B, Grof P, Baastrup RC, Schow M: Lithium prophylaxis in recurrent affective disorders. Br J Psychiatry 116:604, 1970
10. Baastrup PC, Poulson M, Schow M, Thomsen K, Amdisen A: Prophylactic lithium: double blend discontinuation in manic depressive and recurrent depressive disorders. Lancet 2:326–330, 1970
11. Schildkraut J: Catecholamines and classification of depressions. Presented to World Psychiatric Assn, Biological Psychiatric Section, Munich, October 1974
12. Sachar E: Psychiatric disturbances associated with endocrine disorders. In Reiser M (ed): American Handbook of Psychiatry, Vol 4. New York, Basic Books, in press
13. Sachar EJ, Juter S: Unpublished study, 1972
14. Fras I, Litin EM, Pearson JP: Comparison of psychiatric symptoms in carcinoma of the pancreas with those in some other intra-abdominal neoplasms. Am J Psychiatry 123:1553, 1967
15. Goodwin FK, Ebert MH, Bunney WE: Mental effects of reserpine in man. In Shade R (ed): Psychiatric Complications of Medical Drugs. New York, Raven, 1972, pp. 73–101

Chapter 7

Hypochondriasis

Norman Altman

INTRODUCTION

Hypochondriasis has been relegated to a "no man's land" in medicine. A syndrome of psychogenic etiology and somatic presentation, its understanding and treatment are seen by neither the psychiatrist nor the internist as lying within his area of specialization. This is reflected in the relative absence of the subject in the literature and in training programs. The internist feels frustrated, deceived, and angry when his diagnostic efforts convince him that the patient's complaints have no organic basis and all attempts at symptomatic relief fail. The patient's persistent and often hostile demands for treatment only increase when they are dismissed as psychological. Of the few who accept evaluation by a psychiatrist, still fewer are seen as motivated for treatment and able to think of their problems in psychological terms. Psychiatrists usually find it difficult to understand the behavior of these patients, which is unlike the usual psychopathology they see. They sympathize with the internist but have little to offer.

The discussion of the organic brain syndromes in Chapter 4 deals extensively with the inability of either psychiatrists or internists to integrate the behavioral and physical aspects of these disorders into a holistic understanding and management of the patient. This is also true in hypochondriasis, where the patient's need for medical treatment is one that most psychiatrists feel unable to fulfill, just as most internists feel neither capable of nor interested in treating a psychological disorder.

Hypochondriasis, like the organic brain syndromes, presents psychiatrists and internists with a fertile area for collaboration. Clearly, both have a great deal to offer each other toward an understanding and rational management of these patients.

CLASSIFICATION

Until its inclusion under "Hypochondriacal Neurosis" in the most recent revision of psychiatric nomenclature,[1] hypochondriasis was not an official diagnostic entity. It was broadly defined to include any excessive preoccupation with bodily function and, as such, was considered a secondary symptom appearing in many psychiatric disorders. Even the classical, fully developed syndrome to be considered in this chapter has been seen as part of another disorder, as a manifestation of depressive illness. Lesse[2] sees hypochondriasis as a "masked depression" and its symptoms as "depressive equivalents." In a study of 100 patients with hypochondriasis, mainly referred from medical sources, he found that 69 percent had been ill for more than two years and 16 percent for more than ten years. There was a long history of unsuccessful medical treatment and an unremitting course. Patients in this group were described as proud of their suffering, displaying much overt anger, and overbearing in their attempts to control their environments. Depression was diagnosed on the basis of positive responses to questions about hopelessness and material that implied diminished self-esteem. Lipsitt also focuses on depression as the primary problem in hypochondriasis[3] and divides the group into subtypes of depression,[4] although most of the patients described demonstrated neither a depressive syndrome nor a therapeutic response to traditional treatments for depression. Indeed, Lipsitt suggests an altogether different approach to the treatment of hypochondriasis. Dorfman[5] considers hypochondriasis a defense against depression, where the affect is displaced onto somatic concerns so that a "masked depression" exists.

It would seem that this exaggerated use of the concept of "masked depression" is counterproductive. The clinical features described: the long, unremitting course of the illness, the fact that the patients studied did not respond to treatment for depression, and their characterization as overtly hostile and proud of their suffering, do not support the diagnosis of depression. It would, instead, argue for a separate entity and the need to differentiate hypochondriasis from other psychiatric syndromes, including depression, in which somatic complaints play a secondary role. To say that a phobia is a "masked anxiety" would be true in the sense that the symptom results from conflict resolution that avoids anxiety, but it would not be helpful to our understanding of the conflict or to the treatment of the disorder. However, that hypochondriasis represents an alternative to depression may indeed be true and should enter into our considerations of dynamics and treatment.

DIAGNOSIS AND CLINICAL DESCRIPTION

The term hypochondriasis will be used here to refer to a chronic condition dominated by preoccupation with bodily function and an unshakable belief that physical illness is present. This is accompanied by vague, shifting somatic complaints markedly exaggerated in relation to physical findings and not significantly relieved by traditional medical treatment. This preoccupation replaces interest in external objects, but regressive relationships exist based on illness and suffering.

The physician should be alerted to this diagnosis when confronted with a patient whose history includes multiple work-ups with insignificant findings, who is unwilling to talk of his life aside from his symptoms, and where the patient dwells on and seems proud of suffering and self-sacrifice. A hostile, provocative attitude, demanding yet disparaging the physician's abilities, will often be present.

Although hypochondriacal patients start their careers with visits to physicians in private practice, in time most find their way to the clinics of general hospitals, typically organized along specialty lines and where each patient does not have a primary physician who is responsible for his overall care. These are patients with urgent complaints and a history of unsuccessful medical care for a variety of symptoms. Complaints in hypochondriasis may focus on any part of the body, although its name derives from the hypochondria, the subcostal abdominal region at first thought to be the focus of pathology. Symptoms related to gastrointestinal function remain the most frequent, followed by those related to the musculo-skeletal system. Symptoms are often vague, shifting, and multiple. Onset of the illness is often related to loss—of either a significant relationship, job, or other sources of self-esteem.

Ordinarily, patients need to be drawn out with careful questions to obtain a medical history. "The hypochondriac comes in, takes over the interview, and knows all there is to be known. He pours out everything he wants to say and does not allow the intrusion of the physician's knowledge and training."[6] He avoids talk of relationships or emotional problems and shifts to somatic complaints. The patient incriminates innocent organs, willingly submitting to and even demanding life-threatening procedures. He usually appears healthy and shows a lack of concern in the "organ recital" he gives. He is overly critical of doctors he has seen and often blames past procedures for current symptoms. At the same time, he disparages doctors who have found nothing wrong. He believes that, so far, no physician has understood his illness. When the clinical work-up shows no organic pathology to account for the type or degree of symptomatology, the patient will respond to this reassurance with anger and an increase of complaints, insisting on further work-up. The doctor–patient relationship then becomes mutually hostile. The patient accuses the doctor of being incapable or incompetent to relieve his suffering, and the doctor intimates that the patient is lying about his symptoms or is emotionally disturbed.[7] Referrals to psychiatrists are rarely followed up by the patient,[3] and attempts to persuade the patient that he needs to come only infrequently for a check-up lead, paradoxically, to increased clinic or emergency room visits. Usually, referral to another clinic follows. Before long the patient may be attending several clinics in the same hospital, and may even be secretly attending clinics at other hospitals as well. At times a physician becomes convinced that further work-up is necessary, and hospitalizations and surgical procedures are not infrequent. Repetitive, extensive investigations will usually show some abnormality, however minor, in anyone. The hypochondriac often responds to such a positive finding with a feeling of vindication and a demand for cure.

Typically, such a patient has poor relationships outside the clinic, and those he has are based on his illness and suffering. Indeed, he takes pride in his long history of suffering and his feeling he has been let down by others for whom he made sacrifices. Despite his lack of enjoyment in life, he is not depressed, for he sees his limitations as imposed upon him. Difficulties in relationships or work, a need to be cared for, angry feelings are all seen as justified by the hypochondriac's sacrifices or symptoms, whereas the depressed person experiences his inabilities to meet his standards as due to a lack in himself.

After some time, usually several years, these patients become known as "thick file cases," "problem patients," or "crocks," and their care is referred to as "psychoceramic medicine." They exhaust both the clinical facilities and emotional reserve of the medical staff. Yet the patients, too, have a sense of frustration as they work at cross-purposes to the staff and are forced to continue their symbolic search for care in an environment in which they truly are misunderstood.

Epidemiological studies are rare because of the vagueness of the definition of this disorder in the past and its lack of differentiation from other syndromes in which somatic complaints occur. In most studies[2, 4, 8] and in ours in the Montefiore Hospital medical clinic,[9] hypochondriacs were almost all women, usually postmenopausal, whereas Pilowsky[10] found a more equal sex distribution. Hollingshead and Redlich[11] found that an increased concern with bodily sensations was most common in socially and economically deprived classes.

DIFFERENTIAL DIAGNOSIS

Hypochondriasis must be differentiated from other psychogenic conditions in which somatic symptoms may be present. These include depression, conversion reaction, psychophysiological reaction, obsessive neurosis, schizophrenia, malingering, and somatic complaints of a minor and occasional nature.

Depression. Many people with depression are not aware of it. Unconsciously they dissociate affect from content and displace the affect onto physical concerns. Some somatic symptoms, such as anorexia, insomnia, constipation, and diminished sexual interest, are common in depression. Guilt may lead to thoughts of having cancer, venereal disease, and so forth, which may be as unshakable as the need for punishment. That people with these symptoms often come first to a medical clinic is well documented in studies of patients with marked somatic complaints unrelated to physical findings. Between 20 percent[12] and 50 percent[10] were found to have depressive illness. Depressive illness, however, differs from hypochondriasis in several ways. It does not have an unremitting course of years' duration, but is often a discrete, though often recurrent, illness lasting up to six to twelve months without treatment. Patients with depressive illness report their symptoms and suffering with feelings of intense sadness, despair, and a feeling that they are deserved. Unlike the hypochondriac, expression of anger is typically inhibited, feelings of worthlessness are dominant, and dysphoric mood does not change much in response to those around them.

Both conversion reaction and psychophysiological reaction may occur alone or as part of other psychiatric syndromes, including hypochondriasis.

Conversion reaction. Conversion reaction, like hypochondriasis, presents somatic symptoms not related to underlying organic pathology but involving loss of function usually not adhering to anatomical reality. The symptom tends to be localized and symbolically represents longed-for but prohibited wishes. In the patient with conversion reaction, apparent loss of function as extreme as blindness or limb paralysis causes little concern ("belle indifference"), unlike the hypochondriac whose demands for relief are most urgent.

Psychophysiological reactions. The term psychophysiological reactions is used here to refer to psychophysiological reactions involving symptoms which are concomitants of anxiety rather than a defense against it. Actual pathological function, usually autonomic, is an acute or chronic manifestation of anxiety, and bodily complaints are related to this. Often the patient is not aware of this connection and anxiety is displaced from the real cause to the symptoms, with resulting fear and misinterpretation that the symptoms denote serious medical illness. These patients are often helped by explanations and reassurance. A common example is the symptom picture related to hyperventilation and including shortness of breath, paresthesias, and syncope.

Obsessional neurosis. Obsessional neurosis may take the form of fear of illness or disease. Preoccupation will be with ritualistic behavior that will protect against such contamination, and this may severely limit the patient's ability to function. The patient is constantly on the alert, often with great attention to bodily function, to be sure his protective measures have been successful. When anxiety breaks through these defenses, the patient may come to the physician. Usually, these patients are well controlled, and rarely become angry except when forced to change their routine.

Schizophrenia. In certain stages of schizophrenia, somatic concerns, often bizarre, are common. In very early stages a generalized withdrawal from external interests frequently results in an increase of attention to bodily feelings and function. Patients may complain of a variety of symptoms, often related to pains and weakness, and may be treated for these or may be thought to be hypochondriacs. As the psychotic process develops over a period of days or weeks, these somatic symptoms diminish and may be replaced by delusions related to the body—that the body is "rotting" or the stomach is "full of worms," for example. Conviction of disease may be part of the patient's delusions of persecution. Initial schizophrenic episodes in younger people appear with more extreme and widespread disruptions in functioning than are seen in hypochondriasis.

Malingering. Malingering, the conscious simulation of illness, is usually associated with localized symptoms and feigned positive findings in physical examinations, which are difficult to duplicate consistently. However, secondary gain, generally financial, and frequently apparent in the malingerer, is usually absent in the hypochondriac. On the other hand, the hostile demandingness and preoccupation with the body that characterize the hypochondriac are unlikely to be present in the malingerer.

By far the largest group of people with functional or psychogenic somatic symptoms are those Turnbull[13] terms "temporary hypochondriacs"— persons who develop symptoms and a fear or conviction of illness only occasionally and when under stress. Mechanic[14] notes that British and American morbidity surveys have shown that "three of four people have symptoms in any given month for which they take some definable action such as use of medication, bed rest, consulting a physician and limiting activity." People who develop in a cultural setting in which it is permissible to seek help for emotional distress are likely to do so. Where this has been discouraged, a person may seek help for such distress through the acceptable expression of somatic complaints. This occasional focus on and misinterpretation of bodily sensations that would normally be regarded as trivial and that might temporarily serve to mollify a feeling of failure, avoid a feared situation, or justify seeking comfort from others does not fit our definition of hypochondriasis. It lacks the chronicity, unshakable conviction of illness, and regressive external relationships that are characteristic of true hypochondriasis.

Finally, the hypochondriac need not be a constant medical patient, although those who are form the basis for our attention, study, and difficulties in management. Many maintain their conviction of illness without going to doctors, if their environment responds in a need-fulfilling manner, that is, if relationships are stable and controlled and self-esteem is maintained. Only when these are threatened is the hypochondriac likely to turn to the medical setting or to present severe management problems when forced to go to the clinic or hospital by actual organic illness.

DYNAMIC CONSIDERATIONS

Cowen[15] considers hypochondriasis a psychosis in which the goal of thinking and behavior is to maintain delusions of persecution and grandeur, and others[16] support the official designation of hypochondriasis as a neurosis explainable in terms of conflict, anxiety, and defense. But hypochondriasis can best be understood if it is viewed as a transitional state between neurosis and psychosis.[4, 6, 17] Of central importance is the general withdrawal of emotional investment in external objects and displacement of it onto the self as object. The body becomes a substitute for interpersonal relationships and this severe regression distinguishes hypochondriasis from the neuroses. Ordinarily the hypochondriac does not have as pervasive a break with reality or as generalized an impairment of ego functioning as that seen in the psychotic. Hypochondriac-like states are common not only at the start of the schizophrenic process[17] but also in terminal stages of illness,[18] and this is consistent with the withdrawal from external objects and regression that occur in these conditions. Norton[18] has offered convincing evidence that somatic preoccupation in terminal illness may be avoided when a strong external relationship is maintained.

Mally and Ogston[8] described the women they studied as involved in an ambivalent, masochistic relationship with their mother (or mother surrogate). These women felt misused and angry, having tried in vain to win love and care by doing and being good. Their father was never close, but was fantasized as the longed-for magical supplier of unending care. In their later relationships, no man could ever approach this ideal. These patients' focus on illness in the medical setting was seen as a reenactment of the ambivalent relationship with their mother.

In our study of hypochondriacal patients in the medical outpatient department,[19] as in Lipsitt's,[4] we were most impressed by the prevalence of masochistic character features and the defensive use of somatization. Also striking was the poverty of relationships outside of the hospital and the use of illness in the service of maintaining gratifying, though extremely ambivalent, transference relationships with medical personnel. Both psychiatric interviews and ratings on the Hamilton Scale confirmed the absence of depression. Hypochondriasis served the ego function of conflict resolution by allowing these patients to express impulses, primarily dependency and anger, without loss of self-esteem. This was possible, however, only because their conviction of being ill justified their impulses and perceived limitations and minimized conflict. It is essential to realize that the hypochondriac is not consciously deceiving anyone. Only his belief in his illness protects his self-esteem. If the doctor validates and supports this conviction, the patient can avoid anxiety and depression and maintain regressive relationships. In our society no one blames a sick person for not doing his job or for being more demanding.

DIAGNOSTIC TYPES

Our study of hypochondriasis suggests a division into two groups: (1) the masochistic, hostile patient denies his dependency needs and must defend against guilt about his anger and dependency; (2) the less common clinging, demanding patient accepts authority and wants passive, childlike relationships with authority figures.

Type I

The "masochistic-hostile" hypochondriac has regressed to an anal-sadistic stage in which conflict with parental authority centers about control of bodily functions. There is a need to repress aggressive impulses as the price he must pay for love and care. This patient's dominant defenses are reaction formation, projection, and denial. His hostile and sadistic impulses toward his parents are displaced onto organ representations and are also projected onto parent substitutes. He then perceives his anger as a justified response to unfair treatment. Nevertheless guilt remains, though repressed, it motivates a need for suffering in the form of symptoms and the expectation of "something worse to come." These patients dwell on the sacrifices and suffering in their life. Often there is a history of self-sacrifice for a parent or the patient's own family, which previously served to justify the patient's limitations and demands. These patients are able to maintain relationships and self-esteem until a disruption occurs, such as the death of a parent or a child's growing independence. Sickness becomes another form of self-sacrifice through which the patient seeks to maintain his psychological equlibrium.

Mrs. W., a healthy-looking, well-dressed, 63-year-old divorcee, has a seven-year history of severe abdominal complaints which have eluded diagnosis. Her clinic and ER visits have become more frequent in the last two years; and there has been a marked increase in pain in the last ten days. The patient brings stools to the ER almost daily to show that they are bloody, although she has been told repeatedly that they are not.

She is obviously angry because the clinic staff treat her "like I'm not really sick." She is controlling and manipulative, and actively seeks an exclusive relationship with the physician. She dwells upon her life-long sacrifices for her family, her own suffering, and emphasizes how good she's always been.

MEDICAL HISTORY

Repeated work-ups over the years in a GI clinic resulted in surgery for excision of a rectal polyp four years ago, but there have been no other positive findings. Complaints of unbearable right upper quadrant pain have persisted over the past two years, without response to symptomatic treatment or reassurance.

PSYCHOLOGICAL HISTORY

Mrs. W. grew up in a family in which only the boys were valued. She had been forced to drop out of school to earn money so her brothers could go to college, and so her younger sister could finish school. However, she continued to live with her parents even after her sister had married and they were no longer financially dependent on her. After her father died, fifteen years ago, she had felt it was her "duty" to take care of her "senile" mother. And seven years ago she felt it was her "duty" to leave the "good" job she had held for twenty years, because her mother could not be left alone. Her mother died two years ago.

Mrs. W. feels her mother never appreciated her efforts or the sacrifices she made. She is angry with her brothers, who want to help her now, but were never there when she needed them, and she is jealous of her sister. Now she "only lives for" her sister's children.

MEDICAL-PSYCHOLOGICAL CO-VARIANTS

Mrs. W. had been in excellent health until she was "forced" to leave her job to take care of her mother full-time. This decision coincided with the onset of her abdominal pain, which has persisted. The increase in clinic and emergency room visits two years ago coincided with her mother's death; at this point the patient was afraid that, like her mother, she had had a cerebral infarct. Finally, her complaints of increasingly unbearable pain coincided with the death of her nephew, who was killed in an accident ten days ago. However, the patient denies that there was any connection between these events and her symptoms.

A variation of the Type I patient is the patient who is still primarily involved in a self-sacrificing relationship, and whose physical illness provides a means of escape from the situation when her anger becomes too intense. Here, the plea is not just for validation of symptoms but also for temporary removal from the ambivalent relationship in a manner that absolves the patient of guilt.

Miss O., a 41-year-old single woman, has a six-year history of extensive clinic use and several hospitalizations, the last one six months ago. Her main current complaint, of right flank pain, has taken on a greater urgency in the last several weeks, and she has demanded hospitalization once again.

MEDICAL HISTORY

Miss O. has had numerous GI series, intravenous pylograms, and sigmoidoscopies, and has undergone various surgical procedures involving the G-U tract. Hospitalization six months ago for investigation of a possible compressed lumbar disc disclosed no organic pathology. In the past month she has been seen in four different clinics. In the last year she has had negative work-ups for renal tumor, sigmoid tumor, and TB.

MEDICAL-PSYCHOLOGICAL CO-VARIANTS

Miss O. was well and working until six years ago when she started to devote full time to caring for her chronically ill, elderly mother. Shortly thereafter Miss O. had her first operation, and she attributes all of her physical troubles since to that and subsequent surgery. Doctors caused her problem; then they refused to give her the care she needed. There was an obvious parallel when she spoke angrily of sacrificing her life for mother who gave nothing in return. Although she complains of her inability to tolerate her mother's demands, she has never thought of leaving her. Recently, as they have from time to time in the past six years, her mother's demands have become unbearable, but the patient makes no connection between this, her consequent anger, and her increasing symptoms and demands for hospitalization. She attributes her lack of close relationships throughout her life to the demands of work and her sacrifices for her mother.

Type II

Type II is the "clinging, dependent" hypochondriac. This patient's regression is to a passive, oral stage, at which an expression of discomfort is expected to bring prompt parental care. Relationships are anaclitic, with almost complete dependence on a mother substitute, and feelings of helplessness to control or effect need fulfillment predominate. Ego function is not sufficiently developed to meet life's challenges. This poor ego functioning and a tendency to form rapid, undiscriminating transference relationships are evidence of a borderline state in these patients. They usually present with a multiplicity of vague symptoms as a way to communicate their need to a physician or nurse in whom they hope to find a good parent. However, they tend to see the parent substitute as uncaring, like the parent he replaces, and will often provoke rejection. These patients are often isolated and lonely, and their symptoms start or increase upon threatened or real loss of a parent substitute. Complaints do not have the same angry quality as with the "masochistic-hostile" patient. Visits to the doctor or clinic are seen as social events, and the patient will loudly proclaim his long association with the doctor as if claiming a family relationship.

> Miss U., a 28-year-old single woman, is regarded by the clinic nurses as their most difficult patient. She has come to the clinic and emergency room several times a week for the past year with multiple symptoms, usually abdominal, but recently related to severe shoulder pain. Neither medication nor reassurance has helped, and her complaints have taken on the quality of accusations which are leveled against the staff for not caring for her adequately. She has a childlike dependence on two of the clinic nurses.

MEDICAL HISTORY

Miss U. was healthy until she was 18 years old; she attributed the onset of her abdominal pains to the onset of her menses at that age. At the age of 19, persistent pain on her left side led to an operation for an ovarian cyst, followed a year later by an operation for a "misplaced appendix," and a cholecystectomy when she was 22.

The patient had come to our medical clinic because she felt that conservative treatment of continued abdominal pain at another hospital hadn't helped. In the past year, extensive work-ups, including one for porphyria, have shown no organic pathology. She has been seen in the GI, orthopedic, urology, and allergy clinics.

PSYCHOLOGICAL HISTORY

Miss U. was brought up in foster homes and did not meet her mother until she was 13, when she discovered that her mother had kept her two younger sisters. She then lived with her mother for a year, until her mother remarried. The patient could not bring herself to move into her stepfather's house. For the past six years she has lived in a home run by the church, but has formed no relationships with her peers. She has stayed away from her mother, who, she feels, has always been ashamed of her and rejected her. She seeks a childlike relationship with the clinic nurses, but sees them, too, as bad mothers who reject her because of her defects, that is, her symptoms.

MEDICAL-PSYCHOLOGICAL CO-VARIANTS

Miss U.'s somatization was pronounced. When we talked about her feelings of rejection by her mother, she cried—but immediately related the crying to increased shoulder pain and substantiated this complaint with demands for relief.

MANAGEMENT

Physicians vary in their desire or ability to manage the hypochondriac, but it seems certain that this will become an even more pronounced problem for physicians as health insurance makes the private and group practitioner accessible to these patients in a way that only clinics are now. Only by understanding the patient's behavior can the physician cope with his own feelings and attempt rational management.

The psychiatrist may be directly involved in the management of the hypochondriac, but more often will be called upon to advise the primary care physician. In either circumstance he must understand that the appropriate approach to the patient is a supportive, sustaining one, rather than an attempt to promote insight or use confrontation to induce the patient to give up his symptoms.

It may be helpful before discussing the supportive approach, to consider a few techniques that are not rational and do not work. There is a great tendency for the doctor to ignore the emotional illness and engage in prolonged work-ups, referrals, and procedures without ample indications. Often, a considerable amount of time elapses before the doctor acknowledges the patient's primary emotional problem. But having acknowledged the emotional illness, the doctor's reassurance that nothing is wrong or attempts to persuade the patient that his illness is emotional will only bring about an increase in the patient's symptoms. However, giving a positive organic diagnosis and specific treatment does not cure a hypochondriac either. "There is no medication that will alter the psychological need for illness and no surgery that will cut it out."[20] In all of the above attempts at treatment there is a disparity between the objectives of the patient and those of the doctor. The goal of treatment is to minimize this disparity by allowing the patient to maintain his defense (his illness) with a minimum of suffering and a minimum use of medical services. The general approach is to understand the patient's need and then to listen to his symptoms without challenging them or being seduced into making a diagnosis. If a diagnosis is given, it should imply chronic but benign disease. Initially the doctor can say, "My examination shows there's nothing dangerous going on, but I can understand how miserable these symptoms make you. Many people have such chronic symptoms without the cause ever being found. I can't remove the symptoms, and this may be a burden you'll have to carry for a long time, but I would like to work with you to help diminish your discomfort in any way I can." Aside from this general approach, management of the two types of patients described above can proceed as follows.

Type I

The masochistic patient is controlling and manipulative and engages the doctor in endless battles over drugs, treatment goals, demands for tests, and so forth. If the doctor begins to feel guilty and frustrated, the patient will too and his symptoms will increase. If the doctor can curb his guilt and treatment zeal, he can support the patient's efforts to increase self-esteem through self-sacrifice for his family and in other ways. The doctor praises strength in the face of hardship, but doesn't demand it.

These patients react poorly to drugs unless they are allowed to help in deciding which ones help them most. When mild drugs are given, it should be without hopes for great improvement, though with the idea that they might provide some relief. The patient should always be given a return appointment date and be allowed to help decide on the interval between appointments. These patients stress their independence and ability to suffer and will try longer intervals between appointments. As with drugs, permitting the patient to participate in such decisions minimizes conflict. As a general guideline, the treatment session itself should never last more than twenty or thirty minutes, saving the last five minutes or so for a brief physical examination, taking blood pressure and pulse, specifically checking into symptoms, and renewing of medications, if necessary. Except for the examination, the doctor's role in the treatment session is a passive one, in which he listens sympathetically and at intervals indicates his understanding of how difficult or uncomfortable things must be for the patient. When the patient has done something independent or something to help others, the doctor shows appreciation of his strengths with a statement such as: "It's wonderful that you can do something like that despite the distress you have." The patient's pleasure will be obvious, although he may try to cover it with a rapid switch to a report of symptoms.

As the doctor indicates interest in the patient beyond his symptoms, the patient will talk more and more about other things in his life. Although complaints about symptoms remain, the steam goes out of them. If a session does proceed without mention of the symptoms, it is well for the doctor to inquire about them before the patient leaves. When symptoms increase, with mounting demands that the doctor "do something," the doctor should see this as a reflection of increased anxiety which, in all likelihood, is caused by events outside the treatment, and not feel guilty or slip into an inappropriate active treatment role. The doctor must remain alert to the development of genuine organic illness, but in time he becomes able to detect the difference between an organic symptom and the hypochondriacal one via the quality of reporting.

Type II

In general, the dependent patient is handled the same way as the masochistic patient. However, in contrast to the masochistic patient, the dependent patient accepts the doctor's authority and presents a management problem only when the doctor is seduced into acting the part of the rejecting parent. With these patients the doctor does play the parental role, whereas with the masochistic patient group this would only lead to conflict. With the dependent patient, the doctor must be in full control of decisions about medication and the intervals between visits. When the patient's symptoms increase, it is usually a reflection of his attempt to get the doctor to see him more frequently. The doctor then says firmly that he is well aware of these symptoms, that he knows they are uncomfortable for the patient, but that they present no other threat, and that additional appointments will not help. He sticks to the next scheduled appointment unless there is evidence of crisis in the patient's life outside the treatment. Although the patient may make further attempts to increase the frequency of appointments, as long as the doctor's concern for him comes through, he will accept the limits the doctor sets. The doctor must be firm. A doctor cannot treat these patients if he is afraid that showing a caring attitude will invite demands that he cannot refuse.

The expected course of treatment in both groups will extend over one or two years, and perhaps longer for dependent patients. During this time, although the symptoms may remain, there will not be the extended work-ups, procedures, and hospitalizations which would take place if the routine medical or psychological approach were used. Moreover, the patient's general life functioning will improve, reflecting his increased self-esteem and decreased anxiety. At some point the patient may suggest that he no longer needs to come for treatment. The doctor responds that he will see the patient a few more times and they can then decide. If the patient raises this issue again, and does not experience an increase in symptoms, treatment can be terminated or put on as needed basis.

CONCLUSION

Now, perhaps, we are better able to understand why the hypochondriac becomes resentful when a doctor says he can find nothing wrong with him, and why he finds no solace in such "good news." The essence of effective treatment is contained in the statement: "Never challenge or disparage the symptoms of a hypochondriac."[20] The hypochondriac depends on a conviction of illness in order to keep his defenses intact. What he is really demanding from the doctor is a relationship that will satisfy infantile needs, although these needs are disguised in somatic symptoms. A physician who treats only the symptoms works at cross-purposes to the patient's interests. In hypochondriasis the symptoms are not directly accessible to treatment but can be modified indirectly by a supportive relationship that strengthens the patient's defenses.

There is, as Franklin[21] points out, a need "for a change in medical thinking" and for the elimination of "diagnosis by exclusion" in psychogenic illnesses. A further institutional change is needed specifically for care of the hypochondriac, who cannot be managed in a multispecialty clinic where he does not have his own primary physician. An interesting alternative has been used by Lipsitt,[3] who established an "Integration Clinic" with a psychiatrist as part of the staff of the medical outpatient department. Utilization of the same staff and environment the hypochondriacs were use to did not threaten their defenses based on illness, as had attempts to refer these patients to psychiatric settings.

Further exploration of management methods is certainly indicated. The study by Mally and Ogston,[8] in which hypochondriac "untreatables" were seen in a weekly group over a period of three years, offers great promise. Although these patients' competition, demandingness, and manipulative behavior within the group changed little, there was some symptom relief, reduced need for medications, greater social interaction outside of the group, and a marked decrease in clinic and hospital use. Attempts are now under way to institute this approach in other medical settings.[22]

REFERENCES

1. Diagnostic and Statistical Manual of Mental Disorders, 2nd ed. Washington, DC, American Psychiatric Assn, 1968, p. 41
2. Lesse S: Hypochondriasis and psychosomatic disorders masking depression. Am J Psychother 21:607, 1967
3. Lipsitt D: Medical and psychological characteristics of "crocks." Psychiatry Med 1:15–27, 1970
4. Lipsitt D: The rotating patient. J Geriatric Psych 2:51–61, 1968
5. Dorfman W: Hypochondriasis as a defense against depression. Psychosomatics 9:248–251, 1968
6. Cohen A: The physician and the crock. In Usdin G (ed): Practical Lectures in Psychiatry for the Medical Practitioner. Springfield, Ill, Charles C Thomas, 1966, pp. 22–30
7. Smith JA: Hypochondriasis: symptom or entity. Psychosomatics 11:413–415, 1970
8. Mally M, Ogston W: Treatment of the untreatables. Int J Group Psychother 14:3, 1964
9. Altman N, Strain J, Feuer M: Problem patients in the medical OPD. Unpublished preliminary findings
10. Pilowsky I: Primary and secondary hypochondriasis. ACTA Psychiatr Scand 46:273–285, 1970
11. Hollingshead AB, Redlich FC: Social Class and Mental Illness: A Community Study. New York, Wiley, 1958
12. Kreitman N, Sainsbury P, Pearce K, Costain WR: Hypochondriasis and depression in out-patients at a general hospital. Br J Psychiat 111:607, 1965
13. Turnbull JM: Hypochondriasis. In Bowden CL, Burstein AG (eds): Psychosocial Basis of Medical Practice. Baltimore, Williams & Wilkins, 1974, pp. 73–80
14. Mechanic D: Social psychologic factors affecting the presentation of bodily complaints. N Engl J Med 287:1132–1139, 1973
15. Cowen J: The hypochondrical patient in the physician's office. Ill Med J 139:66–69, 1971
16. Chrzanowski G: Neurasthenia and hypochondriasis. In Freedman AM, Kaplan HI (eds): Comprehensive Textbook of Psychiatry. Baltimore, Williams & Wilkins, 1967, pp. 1163–1167
17. Fenichel O: The Psychoanalytic Theory of Neurosis. New York, Norton, 1945, pp. 261–265, 418–420
18. Eissler KR: The Psychiatrist and the Dying Patient. New York, International Universities Press, 1955

19. Norton J: Treatment of a dying patient. Psychoanal Study Child 18: 541–560, 1963
20. Lyon J: On the Treatment of Hypochondriasis. Univ Colorado, unpublished
21. Franklin LM: The thick file case. NZ Med J 74:253, 1971
22. Vega B, Burros N: Personal communication

Chapter 8

The Problem of Pain

James J. Strain

Of all the clinical problems reviewed in this section, pain is affected most by the limitations necessarily imposed on the content and scope of a primer. For instance, I have made no attempt in this chapter to discuss the myriad etiological agents that can produce pain, e.g., porphyria, trauma, surgical procedures, nerve degeneration, joint capsule deterioration, expanding mass lesions, and the thalamic syndrome. Nor is pain discussed in terms of specific syndromes, such as low back pain, headache, and acute abdominal pain. I have not described the many modalities now available for the treatment of pain—hypnosis, acupuncture, biofeedback, transcendental meditation, and so forth—which have not yet been incorporated into routine hospital care. Rather, my primary goal is to enhance understanding of this symptom, regardless of its cause, in the medically and surgically ill patient, and facilitate its management in the hospital setting. This chapter will focus on the psychological reactions pain evokes in this patient population and examine briefly the nature of psychogenic pain and the problems it presents in differential diagnosis. The discussion of the management of pain, the second focus of this chapter, will center on the knowledge and attitudes of the patient's caretakers toward pain. If these issues are to be understood, they must be preceded by a review of some psychobiological and genetic-dynamic formulations regarding pain.

OVERVIEW

Psychobiological Aspects of Pain

Hoffmeister[1] has summarized the important physical and psychological relationships that exist in pain:

> Pain, in man, may be characterized not only quantitatively by its intensity, but also qualitatively by its nature. First, there is the conscious perception of pain, ie, being aware of painful afferent impulses without appreciable involvement of the emotions. Second, there may be present an emotional component associated with pain, ie, the painful stimulus may produce a change in affect which may be independent of the nature and intensity of the stimulus [see Dallenbach[2] and Auersperg[3]]. This is especially the case when the nature of the pain-producing stimulus is such that it cannot be readily reduced or abolished. . . . The feeling of being helplessly exposed to the painful stimulus may produce marked anxiety and anger.

Pain, then, has three important components: the peripheral stimulus and physical reaction to that stimulus; the central registration of the physical reaction; and the psychological elaboration, if any, of that reaction. In contrast to pain that has an organic basis psychogenic pain has no peripheral stimulus; and there is no central recording of the physical reaction to that stimulus.

Other authors have expanded on this conceptualization of pain. Szasz[4] contends that the symbolization of pain occurs at three levels. First, pain is a signal by which the ego registers the fact that there is a threat to the body's structural or functional integrity. Second, the experience of pain may be shared, that is, communicated to, another individual—"The expression of pain is a fundamental method of asking for help." Third, pain may "no longer denote a reference to the body"—it may denote a complaint, an attack, a retribution, or a warning of impending object loss.

Beecher's study[5] of soldiers injured in war has relevance for our understanding of pain threshold. His subjects showed wide variability in pain tolerance and awareness, and their responses in many instances were quite unrelated to the severity of their lesions. One must conclude from these findings that pain threshold is affected by or related to a combination of biological and psychological factors.

Among those individuals whose response to pain is biologically determined, we would include those patients described by Critchley[6] who have a hereditary absence of response to ordinary painful stimuli. Such patients are characterized by a propensity for traumatic injury, self-mutilation in childhood, and a lack of painful response to infections. The predisposition to pain is also biologically determined, in part. In addition, pain threshold is related to the state of attention and concentration,[7] to the meaning of the pain for the individual, to the body part involved, and to the individual's affective state. For instance, Merskey[8] has reported that anxious patients with persistent pain have a lower pain threshold than depressed patients with persistent pain, and that hypochondriacal patients seem to have the lowest pain threshold.

Genetic-Dynamic Considerations

The central conclusion that emerges from a review of the literature on pain is that the evolving perception of pain is dependent in large measure on the evolving development and experience of the child and on his biological constitution.

Pain is "experienced" by the infant as a catastrophic condition, involving the total self. In the first year of life, hunger and physical discomfort, exposure to strangers, and separation from mother all produce painful feelings of total distress. The classic separation–individuation phase, which normally extends from the sixth to the thirtieth month of life, is probably facilitated by pain, which helps the child to differentiate his body image and other self-representations from the outside world. Frances and Gale[9] have described an experiment in nature that provides compelling evidence in support of this thesis. These authors evaluated an 18-year-old male patient who, from the age of 7 months, had engaged in persistent and strenuous head-banging which they ascribed to the fact that this patient, like those described by Critchley, suffered from a congenital inability to experience pain. Thus, in this instance, head-banging is explained as an attempt on the part of the patient to further body-image formation and self-object differentiation. More precisely, Frances and Gale feel that an absence of pain sensation had limited their patient's capacity to experience a clearly defined body image. Consequently he sought to establish a sense of personal reality by flooding himself with proprioceptive inputs.

Actually, very few cases of congenital absence of pain have been reported in the literature. By and large, the infant experiences intense painful feelings (total distress) in response to a wide variety of noxious stimuli, as noted above. However, with the achievement of body image, and concurrent differentiation between the self and the object world, the child becomes able to tolerate more pain and to localize pain.

On the other hand, although at this stage the child begins to integrate the giving and frustrating aspects of mother, he continues to harbor magical expectations of her infinite capacity to provide relief and protection. Of possible relevance to this hypothesis is Collins' finding[10] that pain threshold and tolerance correlated with the degree to which sixty-two American soldiers had been "protected" as children, as judged by the ratings they received on a Childhood History Questionnaire. Specifically, Collins reported that subjects who were expected (or forced by circumstance) to be "independent" as children were more sensitive to pain in later life. Similarly, other investigators have advanced the proposition that the finding that subjects in lower socioeconomic groups have a lower pain threshold may be related to the fact that these individuals were less protected in childhood, and consequently had an earlier and greater experience with pain. I would extend this proposition to include patients who have been programmed to overreact to pain, as a result of exposure to overwhelming pain in previous illnesses and hospitalizations.

Pain, and physiological pain in particular, may stimulate fantasies associated with past experiences. And such fantasies may give rise to the patient's expressed fears that the pain is "gnawing at my gut," "ripping me apart," "will make my body explode," and so forth. These reactions to pain are referrable to the vicissitudes of various stages of earlier development to which the patient is likely to regress under stress (pain). On the other hand, pain may be linked with unconscious pleasurable sexual fantasies, as is the case in a masochistic perversion.

With the development of the superego, pain comes to be associated with guilt, punishment, and expiation. Normally, guilt is relieved by punishment, and the individual then associates punishment with certain forbidden wishes and acts and automatically tends to avoid them. However, the person who has a persistent sense of guilt may deliberately (albeit unconsciously) seek out emotional or physical suffering to satisfy a need for further ("deserved") punishment.

PSYCHOLOGICAL REACTIONS TO PAIN

Pain as a Psychological Stress

The quantity and quality of the patient's "suffering" depends on his perception of pain, that is, on the nature and degree of the stresses it arouses. Obviously, pain may be experienced at different levels by different individuals. In general, however, it can be said that pain constitutes a major stress in and of itself and, by fostering regression, compounds the seven basic psychological stresses evoked by illness and hospitalization.

When it evokes these stresses, pain may produce a cranky childlike feeling in the patient, with a demand for immediate relief from the doctor, reminiscent of the infant's demand for immediate gratification of his physical needs by the mother. By the same token, the doctor, like the mother, is perceived as "good" if he relieves the patient's pain immediately, and "bad" if he makes the patient wait for relief. Exposure to strange caretakers and separation from the familiar doctor at night and on weekends may produce an increase in the patient's complaints of pain. Many patients are able to tolerate pain better during the day when their "real" doctors and nurses are available than at night when they feel alone and helpless.

The point is that with regression, physical and emotional pain become fused and confused. It follows, then, that the anxieties generated by the perception of pain may, in turn, intensify the pain.

Psychopathological Responses to Pain

On the basis of our knowledge of the genetic dynamics of development, one might hypothesize that certain individuals can be expected to manifest one of many possible psychopathological responses to pain. Engel's description[11, 12] of the "pain-prone" patient is appropriate here. This is a person who repeatedly suffers from one or another painful disability, sometimes with and sometimes without any recognizable peripheral change. We would also include, for example, the patient who elaborates pain so that it takes on symbolic significance, reviving fantasies of damage that far exceed the physiological reality; the patient who uses pain as a means of communication; the patient who uses it as a mode of obtaining love and attention; and the patient for whom pain is a primary source of pleasure.

The apparent ability to tolerate extreme pain may be individually or culturally determined.[13] A man may continue on the job despite severe chest pains because to consciously acknowledge their possible significance is so terrifying that he is forced to deny their presence. Or the same man may suppress his reactions to severe chest pains because of a cultural indoctrination that stressed the importance of rising above discomfort. Patients who must deny their pain as a defense against anxiety, and those who must deny or suppress any weakness or any need to be dependent lest such behavior elicit the disapproval of others or self-condemnation, are likely to manifest a stoicism that may, in fact, have life-threatening consequences.

> A 29-year-old woman experiencing acute abdominal pain refused to acknowledge its existence, or curtail her homemaking activities. Thirty-six hours later she was found unconscious and rushed to the hospital. An emergency laparotomy revealed a ruptured appendix with widespread peritonitis.

PSYCHOGENIC PAIN

Pain is the most common presenting symptom encountered in the medically ill. Moreover, it is usually interpreted by caretakers and patients alike as prima facie evidence of the presence of physical disease.[14]* How-ever, in their study of 182 consecutive general medical patients, Devine and Merskey[16] found that of the group of 137 patients in whom pain was the presenting complaint, 75 percent had no discernible organic disease.†

Psychological processes precipitated by an emotional event may produce pain in several ways. Pain may represent the solution to a psychological conflict, as occurs, for example, in a conversion reaction. The diagnosis of pain as a conversion reaction is contingent on the presence of four specific clinical features: the symptom has symbolic significance and, as such, serves as the resolution of an unconscious conflict, usually sexual in origin; the patient's affective reaction is not in keeping with the symptom; the symptom is not associated with primary physiological structural change; and it does not conform to known anatomical and/or physiological patterns.

Many workers have investigated the relationship between depression and psychogenic pain. According to Lesse,[22] for example, psychogenic pain may mask an underlying depression. Moreover, pain frequently occurs as a somatic symptom in schizophrenic reactions, manic-depressive reactions, hypochondriasis, and so on. The experience of pain may be a sensory hallucination. Or pain may be simulated (for secondary gain).

Because of the protean experience and expression of pain, and because, as mentioned above, the psychological and physical aspects of pain are fused, differential diagnosis of psychogenic pain—as opposed to pain which has a physiological basis—may present a major problem that may defy solution.

The frustration typically evoked in physicians by pain that resists differential diagnosis often leads them to offer a psychological diagnosis by exclusion without necessary and/or sufficient evidence to justify such a diagnosis. Furthermore, physicians faced with this dilemma frequently proceed on the erroneous assumption that placebo will differentiate functional from organic pain, and therefore rely on it as a diagnostic tool. In fact, however, while the power of the placebo is well known, its use in clinical medicine is less certain.[23] Beecher's description[24] of his experimental evaluation of placebo is illuminating in this regard.

> In the beginning, we had no doubt that the various ingenious
> experimental pain methods were useful in man. To our chagrin

---

* Hollingshead and Redlich[15] found that patients in lower socioeconomic groups were more likely than patients in higher socioeconomic groups to ascribe their pain to physical rather than psychological factors.

† The bizarre pain syndromes felt to be of psychogenic origin, eg, Munchausen's syndrome,[17,18] lie outside the scope of this discussion. Nor have we discussed phantom limb pain,[19] despite the frequency with which it occurs (in 12[20] to 33 percent[21] of all patients who have had an amputation).

we were unable to distinguish with the most carefully studied of these methods, the radiant heat method, any difference between a large dose of morphine and a placebo. (And neither was an investigator familiar with this method when he was deceived as to what had been given to the subject.) Our failure was duly reported. It was most unpopular (and so were we), until, eventually, some 14 other groups confirmed our heresy.

Despite Beecher's findings, it is commonly felt that placebo reactors suffer from some form of psychopathology or are "malingering," whereas in fact placebo may lessen or eliminate pain from either psychological or physiological causes. Placebo is frequently as effective as morphine in relieving mild pain, but it is clearly surpassed by analgesics in relieving severe or chronic pain.

Apart from its questionable value as a diagnostic tool, the use of placebo may have a deleterious effect on the doctor–patient relationship. If the patient ultimately discovers that the physician has prescribed placebo, he may feel—with some justification—that he has been "betrayed." The relationship between the nurse and the patient is jeopardized as well. If she believes the patient is being tested for the authenticity of his pain, she will begin to doubt the validity of his complaints.

On the other hand, one can also appreciate the physician's predicament. The clinical example provided below points up the complexity of this problem.

Mr. T., a 52-year-old mechanic, married, and the father of several young children, had injured his right foot at work seven years earlier, at which time he had instituted a lawsuit, which was awaiting disposition. In the years since his accident, the patient had undergone progressive amputations for relief of intractable pain. When he was seen by the psychiatrist, he was scheduled to undergo a chordotomy in a further attempt to relieve his symptoms.

While he was awaiting surgery, Mr. T. verbalized his fear that his pain might be due to cancer. He pressed for surgical correction of his "problem," and continually demanded pain medication. However, his demands for analgesics seemed out of proportion to his manifest distress.

Genetic-Dynamic Considerations

Mr. T. had lost his mother at birth, and was raised by his father and maternal grandmother. At the age of 5 he had been evicted from his father's bed by his new stepmother, and he was subsequently relegated to "third place" by his father when a sibling was born. At the age of 7 his right finger had been severed when he caught it in his father's mower. Mr. T. had contracted tuberculosis when he was 13 years old, and was forced to remain in bed for a year. During this period of enforced bed rest, his father and grandmother were more affectionate and spent more time with him. When he was 17 he learned that a favorite aunt had cancer of the right leg and was expected to die. Contrary to all expectations, however, the aunt survived—after her leg was amputated.

In the years following his accident, Mr. T.'s pain had grown progressively more severe. Two years after his accident, following the birth of his daughter, the patient was unable to leave his house because of pain, and assumed responsibility for the care of his children, while his wife went out to work.

Formulation

The psychogenic contribution to Mr. T.'s pain seemed to lie in his excessive need for affection, to the point where he was willing to offer a body part in return for paternal love. Giving up his leg was a symbolic offering that ensured multiple gains: not only love and attention from his father, but long life, and a means of warding off a more dramatic fantasized amputation–castration. Having his leg cut off also served to foster his identification with his beloved aunt. (Identification with his aunt also meant that if he had the "bad" leg removed, he would not die of cancer either.) Most important, his repeated surgeries legitimized the passive-dependent posture that had proven effective earlier as a mode of getting love and attention from his father. These longings, which had been shaped and intensified by the early death of Mr. T.'s mother and the birth of his daughter, were further reinforced by the prospect of receiving financial compensation for his injury.

THE MANAGEMENT OF PAIN

The symptom of pain challenges the physician's competence as a diagnostician and healer. Moreover, the physician's inability to manage pain compromises his relationship not only with the patient but with the hospital staff and the patient's family, who constantly beseech him to "do something." Under such pressures, he may feel compelled to transfer, overtreat, undertreat, abandon, or blame the patient for not responding to his ministrations. Therefore, when assessing pain in the medically ill patient, the psychiatrist should evaluate the stress the patient places on the doctor, for this may well be a determinant of the patient's response to analgesics.

The insufficient utilization of analgesics for pain, especially in the terminally ill, has been a frequent theme in the recent literature. For example, Marks and Sachar,[25] reporting data gathered from 37 medical inpatients, and from questionnaires sent to a representative group of 102 house doctors in New York teaching hospitals, found that the doctors surveyed subscribed to the belief that patients should be pain-free. Yet, despite the fact that their doctors had prescribed analgesic regimens, 32 percent of the patients studied continued to experience severe discomfort, and 41 percent were in moderate discomfort. Marks and Sachar attribute these findings to the fact that the doctors in their sample underestimated the effective dose range of the analgesic drug prescribed (meperidine), overestimated the duration of its action, and exaggerated the danger of addiction for medical patients receiving this drug in a therapeutic dose range (50 to 150 mg every two to three hours).

> Mr. A., who was 36 years old, 6 feet 6 inches tall, and weighed 250 pounds, was hospitalized for the third time for surgical excision of a pilonidal cyst. The patient was given 75 mg of meperidine every four hours for his severe pain. However, he rang for the nurse every three hours to demand additional pain medication, only to be told to "try to hold out for a little longer."
>
> Mr. A., who was forced to lie on his stomach, became increasingly anxious. The staff attributed his failure to respond to pain medication to his panic and discomfort, and placed a request for a psychiatric consultation for the patient.

Obviously, this was not a therapeutic dose range for a man this size who was suffering from this kind of physical disability, nor was pain medication administered frequently enough to reduce his distress.

At times, however, this deficit in patient management (ie, the underuse of analgesics) extends beyond the physician's lack of knowledge of the effective dose range of a specific drug for a given patient, the duration of its action, or its addictive properties. Rather, it can be speculated that the real obstacle to the appropriate administration of pain medication lies in various unconscious fantasies that may be operative in the physician. These would include, for example, his self-image as an omnipotent healer who should be "sufficient medication" for the patient, his unconscious wish to hurt, and his fear of making the patient dependent on a pleasurable substance—and on the administration of a pleasurable substance—which is a projection of his own fear of becoming dependent in the same sense.

On the other hand, physicians who find it difficult to deal with a suffering patient may tend to overuse analgesics.

> Mrs. F., age 45, was dying of breast cancer. On her physician's orders, she was given analgesics every four hours to keep her comfortable. They served that purpose; however, this medication also induced apathy and a semicomatose state in the patient that precluded meaningful contact with her family. The drug was not an effective substitute for the reassurance and support she might have received from such contact.

The deficit in the management of Mr. A. was clearly due to a lack of pharmacological knowledge. But the deficit in the care of Mrs. F. must be ascribed to more complex factors. In all probability, the overprescription of analgesics in this instance was due to the physician's reluctance to become involved with his terminally ill patient. Witnessing her suffering would make him vulnerable to his own conflicts about suffering and dying. The excessive use of drugs was the physician's defense against such vulnerability.

Of course, the overuse of analgesics may be due to other factors. In the case described below, the physician was motivated by a genuine sympathy for his patient and a desire to ease the patient's plight.

> Mr. Z., a 24-year-old brakeman, suffered from severe sickle cell anemia, complicated by a previous myocardial infarction and recurrent painful thrombophlebitis. The patient was dependent on intramuscular injections of talwin, self-administered several times daily, and called his doctor three or four times a week to make sure he would receive his medication. Even unrelated painful physical symptoms precipitated a panic in Mr. Z.
>
> Mr. Z. was demanding, controlling, and aggressive with the staff, to the point where they found him intolerable. In contrast, Mr. Z.'s physician sympathized with him and was able to tolerate his frequent telephone calls and constant demands for drugs. In fact, Dr. L. felt that his permissive attitude was in keeping with his function as a physician caring for a patient with a potentially fatal illness. He was convinced that he would be "hurting" Mr. Z. if he were not consistently available to him, or denied him his medication on an as needed basis.
>
> According to the patient, he was living on "borrowed time," and was able to live with his serious illness only because of "God's good will—and the doctor's drugs. I might die tomorrow. If I have a pain, it might be my last, because pain affects my heart."

Formulation

In addition to his physical stress, this patient manifested a great deal of psychological stress, which was elicited during the interview. His anxiety about dying, separation, bodily damage, and not being able to work and function as a husband were all exacerbated, and were communicated through pain. The patient sought relief from these stresses by asking for medication, which necessitated longed-for contact with his doctor. In other words, the patient fantasized the physician as his "lifeline," and the doctor, who was really trying to comfort his patient, fulfilled this fantasy, but thereby increased the patient's anxiety. For to the patient this meant that the doctor, too, believed that if he were not constantly available to him, the patient would, in fact, die.

Management

The patient's anxieties had to be dealt with by psychological intervention, that is, exposure and clarification of his fantasies. At the same time, the doctor had to be shown that he was unwittingly increasing the patient's anxiety by his ready availability, and by making drugs easily accessible to him.

Once the doctor recognized that he was contributing to the patient's problem, he and the psychiatrist worked together to devise a plan to reduce the patient's dependence on drugs (and the "drug-doctor"). Specifically, the patient was told that if he wanted to reach the doctor, he should place the call, cancel it, wait an hour, then place the call again if he still felt compelled to ask him for medication. A parallel plan was set up for the self-administration of drugs. If the patient felt he needed pain medication, he was encouraged to wait an hour, and then reevaluate his need for medication.

Guidelines

Certain general comments should be made with regard to the management of pain.

First, when the source of the patient's pain has not been determined, the pain must be treated with caution, for it may constitute a key indicator of an ongoing process. However, the lack of a diagnosis does not contraindicate treatment within limits to secure freedom from pain.

Second, the physician's overriding goal is not necessarily to eliminate pain. As we saw in Chapter 7, the hypochondriacal patient needs his pain.

On the other hand, when pain is due to or exacerbated by psychological factors, the underlying psychological disorder should be treated where possible. For example, Bradley,[26] who described patients in whom pain and depression occurred concurrently, found that antidepressant therapy often alleviated both the affective disorder and the pain that was a symptom of the affective disorder.

Third, by and large, physicians are not sufficiently aware of the need to prescribe analgesics until either symptom relief or toxicity occurs. Nor does the current use of analgesics reflect an essential awareness that patients vary widely in their response and capacity to tolerate pain.

If his efforts to manage pain are to be effective, the physician must understand that body sugar, level of consciousness, metabolic rates, and pain threshold all affect the responses of a given patient to a given amount of a specific drug. Furthermore, the drug-drug effect (see Chapter 9) must be taken into consideration; that is, medical patients may be taking other drugs that inhibit the action of prescribed analgesics and hypnotics.

Tranquilizers may allay anxiety and produce sedation, but they are not a substitute for analgesics, nor is it certain that they potentiate the analgesic effects of narcotics.[27] On the other hand, the conjoint use of tranquilizers and analgesics for the pain syndromes has been recommended.[28] The rationale for this recommendation is clear. According to Hoffmeister,[1] for example, neuroleptics and tranquilizers reduce the emotional response to pain, while the analgesics reduce the awareness of pain (as well as the emotional response it evokes). With the exception of one phenothiazine, methotrimoprazine (levopromazine), which *is* able to reduce the awareness of pain, substantially larger than usual doses of psychotropic drugs would be required to significantly reduce behavioral responses to pain. We know that the doses of psychotropic drugs required to reduce the response to pain in animals are ten to twenty-five times larger than the required dose of morphine.[28] Furthermore, in both animals and humans, repeated use of some psychotropic drugs, for example, meprobamate and phenobarbital, produces an acceleration over time of metabolic degradation, resulting in a relative decrease in effectiveness of the drugs.

The physician must recognize that the surgical treatment, as well as nerve blockade, may be required if analgesics fail to dissipate pain and if psychopharmacological agents cause toxic manifestations, such as central nervous system respiratory depression.

Fourth, the physician must proceed with the understanding that a regimen that includes medication on an as needed basis may put a burden on patients who are psychologically unable to ask for help.

Fifth, pain is frequently a symptom of the quality of the doctor–patient relationship, and may be expressive of the patient's anxiety, anger at his doctor, and/or feelings of rejection. The painful relationship may be experienced, via regression, as a painful body state, as it was in early infancy. The doctor must see this "fit"; that is, he must recognize the effect of the "drug-doctor"[29] as a crucial determinant of the patient's response to pain. The mere availability of the doctor may act as a potent analgesic. On the other hand, an overly involved or overly controlling doctor (or hospital) may exacerbate the patient's pain. Moreover, the doctor's attitude toward pain medication can markedly enhance or diminish the effect of the drug. The findings derived from a study done at the Massachusetts General Hospital by Egbert and his co-workers[30] of the effect of psychological intervention on morbidity clearly supports this contention. Briefly, a group of patients scheduled to undergo abdominal surgery received preoperative visits by the anesthesiologist the evening before their operation. However, only one-half of the patients in the sample selected for study were given information about the recovery room, the pain to be expected, and the medication that would be made available to them to alleviate their discomfort. The authors report that the patients who did receive such information subsequently required less medication for pain and left the recovery room sooner than did patients in the control group who had not received this information prior to surgery.

Sixth, the patient will be better able to tolerate chronic pain if the seven basic stresses normally evoked by illness and hospitalization are reduced. The innovative program initiated by Saunders[31] attests to the validity of this premise. Furthermore, in terminally ill patients Saunders treats pain with drugs that produce a euphorogenic effect, such as adequate doses of heroin. In my opinion, this approach deserves a trial, especially in the terminal patient who continues to suffer intractable pain, despite all efforts to relieve his suffering by conventional means.

REFERENCES

1. Hoffmeister F: Effects of psychotropic drugs on pain. Proc Int Symp Pain. Paris, Laboratory of Psychophysiology, Faculty of Sciences, April 11–13, 1967, pp. 309–319
2. Dallenbach KM: Pain: history and present status. Am J Psychol 52: 331–337, 1939
3. Auersperg A: Schmerz und Schmerzhaftigkeit. Berlin, Springer-Verlag, 1963, pp. 70–76
4. Szasz TS: Pain and Pleasure. New York, Basic Books, 1957
5. Beecher HK: U.F.A.W. International Symposium on the Assessment of Pain in Man and Animals, Keebe CA, Smith R. (eds). London, Livingston, 1962
6. Critchley M: Congenital indifference to pain. Ann Intern Med 45:737–747, 1956

7. Blitz B, Lowental M: The role of sensory restriction in problems with chronic pain. J Chronic Dis 19:1119–1125, 1966
8. Merskey H: The effect of chronic pain upon the response to noxious stimuli by psychiatric patients. J Psychosom Res 8:405–419, 1965
9. Frances A, Gale L: Proprioceptive body image in self-object differentiation: a case of congenital indifference to pain and head-banging. Psychoanal Q 44(1):107–125, 1975
10. Collins LG: Pain sensitivity and ratings of childhood experience. Percept Mot Skills 21:349, 1965
11. Engel GL: Psychogenic pain and the pain-prone patient. Am J Med 26:899, 1959
12. Engel GL: Guilt, pain, and success. Psychosom Med 24:37, 1962
13. Weisenberg M, Kreindler ML, Schachat R, Werboff J: Pain: anxiety and attitudes in black, white, and Puerto Rican patients. Psychosom Med 37:123–135, 1975
14. Merskey H, Spear FG: Pain—Psychological and Psychiatric Aspects. London, Bailliere Tindall, 1967
15. Hollingshead AB, Redlich FC: Social Class and Mental Illness. New York, Wiley, 1958
16. Devine R, Merskey H: The description of pain in psychiatric and general medical patients. J Psychosom Res 9:311–316, 1965
17. Ford CV: The Munchausen syndrome: a report of four new cases and a review of psychodynamic considerations. Psychiatry Med 4:31–45, 1973
18. Cramer B, Gershberg MR, Stern M: Munchausen syndrome: its relationship in malingering, hysteria and the physician-patient relationship. Arch Gen Psychiatry 24:573–578, 1971
19. Noyes AP, Kolb LC: Psychophysiological, autonomic, and visceral disorders. In Noyes AP, Kolb, LC (eds): Modern Clinical Psychiatry, 6th ed. Philadelphia, Saunders, 1963, pp. 409–411
20. Gillis L: The management of the painful amputation stump and a new theory for the phantom phenomena. Br J Surg 51:87–95, 1964
21. Freese AS: Pain. New York, Putnam's, 1974
22. Lesse S: Atypical facial pain syndromes of psychogenic origin: complications of their misdiagnosis. J Nerv Ment Dis 124:346, 1956
23. Shapiro AK, Struening EL: The use of placebos: a study of ethics and physicians' attitudes. Psychiatry Med 4:17–29, 1973
24. Beecher HK: The measurement of pain in man: a re-inspection of the work of the Harvard Group. In Soulairac A, Cahn J, Charpentier J (eds): Pain. New York, Academic Press, 1968, p. 212
25. Marks RM, Sachar EJ: Undertreatment of medical inpatients with narcotic analgesics. Ann Intern Med 78:173–181, 1973
26. Bradley JJ: Severe localized pain associated with the depressive syndrome. Br J Psychiatry 109:741–745, 1963
27. Keats AS, Telford J, Kurosu Y: "Potentiation" of meperidine caused by promethazine. Anesthesiology 22:34–41, 1961
28. Cahn J, Herold M: Pain and psychotropic drugs. In Soulairac A, Cahn J, Charpentier J (eds): Pain. New York, Academic Press, 1968, pp. 335-371
29. Balint M: The Doctor, the Patient and His Illness, 2nd ed. London, Pitman Medical, 1971

30. Egbert LD, Batit GE, Welch CE, Bartlett MK: Reduction of post-operative pain by encouragement and instruction to patient. N Engl J Med 270:825, 1964
31. Saunders C: The treatment of intractable pain in terminal cancer. Proc R Soc Med 56:195–198, 1963

Chapter 9

Psychopharmacological Treatment of the Medically Ill

James J. Strain

Psychopharmacological drugs are an important tool in the care of the medically ill. Not only can they provide relief from the suffering of anxiety and depression, they can alter agitated or hyperactive states that may be life-endangering. However, the use of these agents, which is complicated enough in the nonorganically ill psychiatric patient, requires very special consideration when they are prescribed for patients who have physical illnesses, and who may be receiving other medications at the same time.

It is generally assumed that psychopharmacological treatment lies within the purview of the psychiatrist, and he is expected to be thoroughly familiar with the indications and contraindications for the use of these drugs in the medical, as well as the psychiatric, patient. Unfortunately, however, segments of this crucial knowledge have not yet been sufficiently emphasized in psychiatric training. My purpose in this chapter is to attempt to fill this gap by providing a brief guide to the use of psychotropic drugs for this special group of patients.

GENERAL CONSIDERATIONS

The psychiatrist's approach to psychopharmacological treatment of the medically ill must be governed by the following considerations:

Several colleagues contributed to the content and concepts presented in this chapter. Among these, I would single out Dr. Norman Altman, in particular. I wish to thank Dr. Altman, as well as Drs. Richard Marks, Alfred Wiener, Hoyle Leigh, Selwyn Juter, Bennett Rosner, Ellen Freeman, and T. George Bidder for their assistance.

First, the psychiatrist must establish whether the disturbed patient can be managed on the medical ward. That is, he must decide whether the transfer of the patient to the psychiatric ward, if indicated, would endanger his physical state, or, alternatively, whether maintaining him on the medical ward would be detrimental to him psychologically.

Second, he must evaluate the patient's medical problem, including the drugs currently being employed for its treatment.

Third, the patient's psychological symptoms, for example, anxiety or depression, agitation, psychotic thinking, must be assessed in relation to his personality and modes of coping with stress, and in relation to the "expectable" responses normally evoked by the stresses of illness and hospitalization.

Finally, the psychiatrist must weigh the possible efficacy of alternate modes of handling the patient's psychological symptoms, such as environmental manipulation and verbal reassurance.

In addition, the psychiatrist who prescribes psychotropic drugs for the medically ill patient must take certain specific issues into account:

1. These agents alter behavior, but do not alter the underlying psychological dysfunction.

2. In removing psychological symptoms, psychopharmacological agents may at the same time reduce or eliminate physical symptoms—pain, vomiting, and so forth—thereby obscuring the patient's organic illness.

3. Certain psychopharmacological agents have significant side effects even when they are taken by nonmedical patients. Their potential danger is greatly compounded when they are taken by patients whose illness may have made them particularly vulnerable to a given side effect. The psychiatrist must make a clinical judgment as to the need for psychological symptom reduction versus the possible side effects of a particular drug, bearing in mind as he makes his decision that the physical damage that can result from agitation or hyperactivity frequently outweighs the possible deleterious side effects of psychotropic agents.

The psychotropic drugs can be classified as follows for practical clinical purposes:

CLASSIFICATION OF PSYCHOTROPIC DRUGS

Categories	*Representative drugs*
Major Tranquilizers	
Phenothiazines	
Promazines	Thorazine
Piperidines	Mellaril
Piperazines	Stelazine
Butyrophenones	Haldol

Categories	*Representative drugs*

Minor Tranquilizers

Benzodiazepines	Librium, Valium
	Miltown

Hypnotics

Barbiturates	
Short-acting	Seconal, Nembutal, Amytal
Long-acting	Phenobarbital
Tertiary acetylenic alcohols	Paraldehyde
	Ethchlorvynol (Placidyl)
Chloral derivatives	Chloral hydrate
Antihistamines	Benadryl
Piperidinedone derivatives	Glutethimide (Doriden)
	Methypyrolon (Noludar)
	Flurazepam (Dalmane)

Antidepressants

Tricyclics	Tofranil, Elavil
MAO inhibitors	Nardil, Parnate, Marplan
	Lithium

Analgesics

	Demerol
	Morphine

INDICATIONS AND CONTRAINDICATIONS

Overuse and Underuse of Psychotropic Drugs

Because the potential hazards of some psychotropic drugs, such as Valium, Librium, and Paraldehyde, are not fully understood, it is possible that they are being used excessively for medical patients. Actually, the minor tranquilizers, which are generally viewed as benign, may cause dependency, withdrawal symptoms, and acute organic brain syndromes. And Paraldehyde, which is also thought to be benign, may be addictive. Other drugs, especially the antidepressants, are prescribed inappropriately, for example, for sadness or grief, rather than for diagnosed depressive reactions. The phenothiazines are not used frequently enough for major behavior disturbances because their dangers are exaggerated.

Mr. H., a 48-year-old lawyer, entered the hospital for open heart surgery. He did poorly after surgery, developed pneumonia, and required a tracheostomy. A psychiatric consultation was requested because of Mr. H.'s acute agitation, confusion, and his paranoid state.

The psychiatrist recommended that the patient be given Stelazine. But after the psychiatrist left, the staff were reluctant to follow his recommendation to administer a phenothiazine, in light of Mr. H.'s recent cardiac surgery and his precarious respiratory status. The decision was made instead to administer Valium 0.20 gms intramuscularly.

A few hours after the consultation, the patient, in his confusion, extubated himself, and by the time it was discovered several minutes later, Mr. H. had suffered severe and irreversible brain damage.

The psychiatrist who is sufficiently conversant with the use of psychotropic drugs will know that the substitution of a piperazine, such as Stelazine, for a promazine, such as Thorazine, will lessen the risk of cardiovascular complications and excessive sedation. In fact, the psychiatrist may even go to an entirely different class of drugs to achieve behavioral control.

Mr. Q., a 56-year-old corporate executive, was restless and agitated the day after he had suffered a massive myocardial infarction, and his mounting anxiety further complicated his physical status: his blood pressure was unsteady, and he had a recurrent arrhythmia. He insisted on getting out of bed in order to urinate standing up, which placed further stress on his heart, and when the nurse tried to restrain him, Mr. Q. became excited and pulled out his intravenous lidocaine drip. He then went into a panic, and ran down the corridor, calling his wife's name. When the nurses and doctors were finally able to catch the wide-eyed, shivering patient and get him back into bed, the nurse could not accurately record his rapid and irregular pulse. Obviously, strong measures were called for to control Mr. Q.'s agitated behavior, but because of his myocardial infarction and rapid pulse, his physician was afraid that phenothiazines would be dangerous. The psychiatrist was able to suggest an alternative. On his recommendation 5 cc of Paraldehyde were administered intramuscularly to each buttock. Shortly thereafter, the patient fell asleep.

Therapeutic Potency

Choice of Drug. The doctor may facilitate therapeutic results by substituting one major tranquilizer, for example, for another. However, the substitute should be selected from another category of the same drug family. Doctors who find Thorazine ineffective frequently make the mistake of prescribing another derivative of the promazine category, such as Sparine, instead of moving to an entirely new category of phenothiazines, such as the piperidines (Mellaril), or piperazines (Stelazine), or to the butyrophenones (Haldol).

Dosage. In general, once the doctor has determined the optimal dosage, that is, the one that achieves a therapeutic result without toxicity, the patient should be maintained on that dosage until maximal clinical improvement has occurred. However, response to a given dose of psychotropic drugs, which is probably constitutionally determined, varies tremendously from individual to individual. To illustrate, when Glassman[1, 1a] used blood level as a criterion of the effectiveness of antidepressants (tricyclics), he found that therapeutic efficacy ranged from blood levels of 30 n gram to 700 n gram percent, with a median value of 200 n gram percent. The dosage administered to achieve these levels varied from 25 mg to 2000 mg a day. Clearly, a dosage that is effective for one patient may be completely ineffective for another. Furthermore, the length of time required to reach the optimal blood level and a steady state for tricyclics may range from 1½ to 20 days.

The effectiveness of antidepressants (tricyclics) may also depend on the concentration of the plasma proteins, which bind some psychotropic agents.[1a] Finally, Prange[2] feels there is an interaction between imipramine and hormones. He found women, but not men, suffering from depressive reactions to be more responsive to imipramine when L-triiodothyronine (T3) was an adjunctive treatment.

Time Required for Drug Effect. Some psychotropic drugs must be administered for several days or weeks before they produce an effect; antidepressants commonly require two or three weeks. Consequently, instituting antidepressant therapy for a medically ill patient who will be hospitalized for less than two weeks would certainly be inappropriate, unless adequate follow-up provision is made for the continued use of the drug, under supervision, after the patient has been discharged from the hospital.

Route of Administration. The route of administration is an important determinant of therapeutic potency. In general, the oral route has the least immediate potency, the intramuscular route has intermediate capacity, and the intravenous route is the most potent. With certain drugs, however, a particular route of administration, while more desirable in terms of therapeutic potency, may be less desirable in terms of dangerous side-effects. For example, when Thorazine is administered intravenously, it has a potent, rapid effect. However, it may induce arrhythmia or lower blood pressure, which may be life-threatening physical symptoms in the medically ill, especially in the cardiac patient. The intramuscular route is less effective, but it is also less dangerous. And the oral route, the least effective, is also the safest. Similarly, the administration of paraldehyde intravenously carries significant danger. On the other hand, the administration of Librium intramuscularly produces a slow, erratic, and incomplete response, compared with the oral route, which produces a rapid, even, and more complete drug response.[3] This is probably true of Valium as well.[4]

Psychopharmacological Approaches to Psychological Symptoms

More specific recommendations for the pharmacological treatment of specific psychological symptoms are given below. T. G. Bidder[5] has suggested five specific approaches to the psychopharmacological treatment of acute agitation, which have as their goal the rapid—and safe—control of such behavior, and the achievement of a maintenance dose that will make the patient manageable. Recommendations are listed for the treatment of anxiety and insomnia as well. The use of antidepressant medication in the medically ill with diagnosed depressive reactions will be discussed only briefly in this context.

SYMPTOM	RECOMMENDED DRUG AND ROUTE OF ADMINISTRATION
Acute agitation	1. *"Pentobarbital Sodium*—5% sterile solution with water, propylene glycol, and alcohol, or freshly prepared aqueous solution. IV or IM, 0.2–0.5 gms. (4–10 ml can be injected immediately IV without delay). Repeat once after 3–5 minutes, or twice if necessary, with this time interval between doses."

2. *"Amobarbital Sodium* (*Sodium amytal*)—5% sterile solution. Only freshly prepared aqueous solutions suitable. IM or IV—0.3–0.6 gm (5–12 ml). Instructions for IV use are the same as for sodium pentobarbital. Ten percent solutions, and consequent smaller injection volumes, can be used IM."

3. *"Paraldehyde*—Retention enema of one part Paraldehyde and two parts olive oil or mineral oil can be given per rectum in doses of 0.5–1.0 ml of mixture per Kg. body weight."

4. *"Chlorpromazine*—Patients who are acutely disturbed, who are relatively young and free from cardiovascular disease, and who are not under the influence of central nervous system depressants such as barbiturates, narcotics and alcohol, may be treated as follows: Initial dose of 25 mg by deep IM injection. In patients in whom satisfactory control of

SYMPTOM	RECOMMENDED DRUG AND ROUTE OF ADMINISTRATION
Acute agitation (cont.)	symptoms is not achieved—and in whom severe cardiovascular (hypotensive) reactions have not occurred—this dose may be repeated one hour later and subsequent IM administration of 50–100 mg may be employed at intervals of 4–6 hours until the patient is quieted. Patients on this regimen should be watched carefully for hypotensive (orthostatic) episodes which are particularly apt to occur in the first hour after injection; the drug should not be used in this manner unless facilities for adequate supervision are available."
	5. "*Stelazine*—Administer 5 mg IM as an initial dose. Monitor blood pressure and sedation. After one-half hour, if there have been no adverse effects, administer an additional 5 mg PO, if possible; otherwise the drug should be given IM. If the patient is not under control within one hour, administer an additional 5 mg. Provided the patient does not become too sedated, he should be maintained on 5 mg q.6h thereafter."
Anxiety	1. *Librium*—5 to 10 mg every four to six hours.
	2. *Valium*—2 to 10 mg every six to ten hours.
	3. *Sodium amytal*—20 to 40 mg every eight to twelve hours.
	4. *Stelazine*—2 mg every six hours.
	Drugs for mild to moderate anxiety are ordinarily given by mouth.
Insomnia	1. *Sodium amytal*—100 to 200 mg.
	2. *Chloral hydrate*—500 mg to 2g.
	3. *Paraldehyde*—3 to 8 ml at bedtime.
	4. *Benadryl*—50 mg.
	5. *Dalmane**—15 to 30 mg.
	The drugs are ordinarily given by mouth.
Depression	The use of antidepressant drugs when a depressive reaction has been diagnosed can only be recommended with reservation. The side effects that commonly occur with these drugs, which are discussed in detail below, may be dangerous and may seriously compromise diagnosis and, therefore, the treatment of medical illness. Consequently, even when it is felt that a depressive reaction will be responsive to antidepressant medication, the use of these drugs requires extreme caution, especially in the elderly, in patients with serious medical illnesses, in patients who have an initial adverse reaction to such medica-

---

* I share Greenblatt's opinion of the advantages of Dalmane: "Although expensive, [Dalmane] permits physiologic sleep, has a low potential for abuse, is an ineffective suicidal agent, and probably does not interact with oral anticoagulants."[4]

SYMPTOM	RECOMMENDED DRUG AND ROUTE OF ADMINISTRATION
Depression (cont.)	tion, and, finally, in patients who are receiving other pharmacological agents that may make antidepressant drugs more toxic. For these patients, the use of electroconvulsive therapy may carry less risk. Precautions apply as well to patients who are on antidepressant medication when they enter the hospital for diagnosis and treatment of a medical illness. The psychiatrist must then decide, in consultation with the internist, whether the drug should be withdrawn and the patient's depression treated by other means. If the decision is made to continue to administer antidepressant drugs, or to administer such medication in progressively reduced dosage, the patient must be watched carefully throughout the course of treatment.

Obviously, these data are an essential part of the doctor's armamentarium. However, they are not sufficient to ensure competent psychopharmacological treatment of the psychological symptoms of his medical patients. He must also be familiar with the clinically important properties of these drugs, which are discussed below.

The Drug-Drug Effect

The drug-drug effect may take two forms. First, the doctor should be aware of the fact that when certain psychotropic agents are given at the same time as other psychotropic agents, both may become less effective. For example, because barbiturates stimulate the production of liver enzymes, they accelerate the degradation of other psychotropic drugs, which then become less effective. Thus, if a depressed patient is given Nembutal for sleep and tricyclics for depression at the same time, both the hypnotic and the antidepressant medication will be less effective.

Other pharmacological agents the patient is receiving may alter the effects of psychotropic drugs. For example, antacids affect the absorption of Thorazine.[7] Moreover, the effects of psychotropic drugs may also be altered by specific illnesses, such as liver diseases that affect metabolic enzyme function, for example, dehydroxylation, demethylation, and deamination.

And, conversely, the psychotropic drugs may alter the effects of other pharmacological agents. For example, Thorazine can inhibit the antihypertensive action of Guanethidine.[8] Ritalin inhibits hydroxylating enzymes, and can markedly increase the effect of a given amount of

Dicumerol. Actually, with Dicumerol there is a biphasic effect: initially barbiturates decrease the effectiveness of a given dose of Dicumerol, but when barbiturates are withdrawn, a rebound phenomenon occurs from decreased enzyme activity, and excessive anticoagulation ensues. There-fore, a change in clotting occurs from adding or subtracting a second drug even when the amount of anticoagulant administered remains constant. In fact, almost all psychotropic drugs are inhibitors of hydroxylating en-zymes. Listed in descending order of their inhibiting capacity, these would include, in particular: (1) Ritalin, (2) tricyclics, (3) phenothiazines, (4) amphetamines, and (5) anticonvulsants.[1]

Side Effects

While the side effects that occur with the antidepressants are not more serious than those produced by the other psychotropic drugs, they are more diffuse and, above all, they are more likely to mimic symptoms of medical and psychological dysfunction. The psychological symptoms that occur with the antidepressants include confusional states, hallucinations, delusions, disorientation, anxiety, and hypomania. In addition, antide-pressant medication may produce such neurological symptoms as numb-ness, tingling, paresthesia, ataxia, tremor, peripheral neuropathy, seizures, alterations in EEG, and tinnitus. The side effects produced by the anti-depressants may, as noted above, mimic medical illness as well, specifically, gastrointestinal disorders, such as constipation, paralytic ileus, anorexia, nausea, vomiting, diarrhea, and abdominal cramps. Or they may produce more diffuse physiological symptomatology, such as fluctuations in weight, dizziness, weakness, fatigue, perspiration, altered blood sugar, and head-ache. Finally, antidepressant medication may produce many of the same side effects encountered with other psychotropic drugs.

Three major cardiovascular side effects are known to occur with the psychotropic drugs. The first is orthostatic hypotension,* leading to symp-toms of syncope, seizures, and tachycardia. This side effect is most likely to occur with Thorazine, less likely with Mellaril, and least likely to occur with Stelazine and Trilafon.† The second side effect, arrhythmia, is par-ticularly likely to occur with Mellaril, especially in patients with myo-cardial infarction. Finally, other EKG changes, such as an increased Q-T interval and a flattened or inverted T-wave, which are usually benign re-polarization disturbances, may occur. When these EKG side effects occur

---

* Certain antidepressants, for example, Parnate, may, in addition to hypotension, cause hypertension under certain circumstances.

† Note that norepinephrine, not epinephrine, should be used to treat phenothiazine-induced shock. Phenothiazines block alpha-adrenergic receptors so that epinephrine has a paradoxical hypotensive effect.

with the phenothiazines (usually during the first week of treatment), they can be eliminated if the drug is discontinued, or if 10 mg of 1-isosorbide dinitrate is given sublingually.

Psychotropic drugs may precipitate two major hepatic side effects: intracellular stasis and biliary stasis. Agranulocytosis is a possible hematological side effect.

Finally, the use of psychotropic drugs can cause glaucoma, urinary retention, rash, and extrapyramidal symptoms.

Solubility

By and large, psychotropic drugs must be converted to water-soluble forms for excretion. Therefore, any medical impairment of that process must be taken into consideration by the doctor before administering these agents. For example, special precautions should be taken with hepatic and renal patients, who have difficulty with metabolism. A drug such as Glutethimide presents a serious problem because it is stored in fat tissue, and dialysis may be ineffective for those who have taken an overdose of the drug.

Overdosage of Psychotropic Drugs

As a rule, psychotropic drug overdose patients are brought to emergency rooms and intensive care units for treatment via the internist. In high doses, many of these drugs can produce central nervous system depression, coma, and death. Davis[9] has given guidelines and has stressed the importance for the psychiatrist to know the special problems of psychotropic drug overdose so that he is conversant with clinical aspects of the management of such patients; he can then relay this information to the internist who is often unfamiliar with this facet of patient care.

Withdrawal from psychotropic drugs, especially if the patient has been on large amounts for some time, may also precipitate a variety of symptoms, such as seizures, anxiety, and vasomotor disorders. For example, if barbiturates are abruptly terminated on the patient's admission to a medical-surgical hospital, profound withdrawal symptomatology may ensue. It is the task of the psychiatrist, therefore, to assist in the development of a satisfactory drug withdrawal regimen.

The Effects of Drugs on the Geriatric Patient

There are special hazards associated with the use of psychopharmacological agents in the geriatric population: (1) Severe toxicity may occur at "ordinary dosages." For example, amitryptyline HCL (Elavil) may be effective in doses of 10 mg, and produce toxic reactions at 25 mg. (2) Aged patients are more vulnerable to hypersensitivity reactions to psycho-pharmacological agents (e.g., dermatological reactions, agranulocytosis, anemias). (3) Because of the heightened susceptibility in this population to cardiovascular and cerebrovascular insufficiencies, psychotropic drugs may lead to congestive heart failure, myocardial infarction, cerebrovascular accidents, syncopal and hypertensive episodes, and to falls resulting in fractures. (4) Paradoxical reactions to drugs often occur in this age group (e.g., barbiturates may cause agitation, disorientation, and aggressive behavior). (5) Long-term side effects of drugs (such as tardive dyskinesias and pigmentary skin and ocular deposits) are common in the aged. (6) The administration of drugs to geriatric patients may complicate or precipitate the appearance of organic disease (e.g., prostatic hypertrophy, angle-closure glaucoma, diabetes, hypertension, congestive heart failure). (7) Finally, in aged patients receiving other drugs at the same time, there is an increased risk of synergistic or potentiating effects.

THE USE OF PSYCHOTROPIC DRUGS WITH SPECIFIC PHYSIOLOGICAL DISORDERS

The fact that certain psychotropic drugs have specific effects on various systems does not necessarily mean that their use is contraindicated. The purpose of this section is to demonstrate that when these drugs are prescribed cautiously, the patient can benefit from their use.

Cardiovascular Disease

Major tranquilizers that are used for major psychiatric disturbances may produce the cardiovascular side effects cited earlier. As noted, Mellaril has been known to precipitate arrhythmias and EKG changes, and Thorazine has a postural hypotensive potential. It is not necessary to use these potentially dangerous drugs, however, with the availability of Stelazine and Trilafon. Stelazine, 2 mg, or Trilafon, 4 mg, administered orally three times a day is often effective for agitation. Stelazine, 5 mg administered intramuscularly, with monitoring of blood pressure, can be used for severe agitation. A minor tranquilizer, such as Librium, 10 mg taken orally four times a day, or Valium, 5 mg taken orally twice a day, can be used for moderate agitation.

Sedation can best be achieved with the minor tranquilizers, chloral hydrate, or Paraldehyde.

Hepatic Disease

In assessing the dangers of using psychopharmacological drugs in patients with liver dysfunction, three separate but related issues must be considered. (1) The drug itself may produce either cholestatic or hepatic cellular defects through an allergic-type reaction. (2) The drug may cause increased hepatic dysfunction, thereby carrying the risk of hepatic coma. (3) Since the defective liver is incapable of metabolizing the drug at a normal rate, there is a danger of drug overdose.

Thorazine, Trilafon, and Compazine caused cholestatic jaundice, which was not dose-related, in approximately 1.5 of the patients studied by Schiff.[10] The jaundice usually appeared two to five weeks after the start of treatment, and ran a benign course after the drug was stopped: symptoms disappeared in two to three weeks without hepatocellular damage. Stelazine and Mellaril carry the least risk of hepatic damage and are therefore the preferred phenothiazines. However, since they are metabolized primarily in the liver, lower and less frequent doses should be given; Mellaril, 25 mg, or Stelazine, 2 mg, should be administered intramuscularly every two hours, with careful monitoring for excess sedation or hypotension, until behavior is controlled, following which the drug should be administered orally. Thus, in summary, although hepatic side effects do occur with the phenothiazines, the rarity of this response should allow the use of psychotropic drugs, including the phenothiazines, when behavioral modification is mandatory.

Cholestatic jaundice can also occur with the minor tranquilizers, although it is rare, and there is no direct toxic effect on the liver. However, since these drugs are also metabolized primarily by the liver, smaller and less frequent doses than usual are required, for example, Librium in a dose of 5 to 10 mg taken orally three times a day, or Valium, 5 mg taken orally twice a day.

In patients with liver dysfunction, sedation should not be achieved by means of the usual drugs. Paraldehyde carries a high risk of hepatic coma, as do the short-acting barbiturates. The long-acting barbiturates are safer, but must be given much less frequently than usual. Chloral hydrate is metabolized mainly by the liver; therefore, its margin of safety is greatly reduced in patients with hepatic dysfunction. Sedation is best achieved with one of the phenothiazines, minor tranquilizers, or antihistamines.

Morphine and Demerol have traditionally been used as tranquilizers, as well as analgesics. Morphine is contraindicated in the presence of liver disease, because it carries a high risk of precipitating hepatic coma. Demerol, on the other hand, bypasses liver function completely and is the safe drug in usual doses.

Renal Disease

Renal impairment has significant consequences for the use of psychotropic drugs: (1) Many drugs are excreted via the kidneys in a pharmacologically active form, which means that there is an increased risk of overdose. (2) The accumulation of toxic metabolic products and electrolyte imbalance may produce an altered state of consciousness. (3) Blood pressure is frequently unstable in patients with renal impairment. Therefore, the potential side effects of Thorazine, for example, sedation and hypotension, take on special significance, and Stelazine would be the preferred drug. With moderate renal impairment, the usual dosages of the phenothiazines are halved. When impairment is severe, dosages are cut to one-third, with careful monitoring to avoid overdose.

With regard to the minor tranquilizers, Valium is the drug of choice because it is fully metabolized nonrenally, and usual dosages can be given. Librium, on the other hand, is excreted in an active form by the kidneys, producing an extended effect.

Sedatives should be used with caution. Phenobarbital (a long-acting barbiturate) is contraindicated because it is excreted by the kidneys in active form. Seconal (a short-acting barbiturate), Paraldehyde, and chloral hydrate are preferred because they are metabolized nonrenally. However, small doses should be given initially to guard against oversedation. Codeine and morphine are not excreted by the kidneys in active form, so usual dosages may be employed, with careful monitoring to avoid oversedation.

Diseases of the Central Nervous System

The main concerns in the administration of psychotropic drugs to patients with lesions of the central nervous system, for example, an intracranial expanding mass lesion, are undue excitation and depression of the CNS. It is also important to avoid interfering with the level of consciousness in cases where obtundation would preclude clinical monitoring.

Of the phenothiazines, Mellaril is least likely to produce extrapyramidal side effects. All the other phenothiazines, and Thorazine, in particular, have been implicated in lowering the seizure threshold, and may produce akathesias, dyskinesias, rigidity, spasms, and dystonias.

Mr. S., a 67-year-old widower, suffered from inanition and slow, purposeless, involuntary movements, which were thought to be due to senile dementia. This diagnosis provided a rationale for the decision to transfer the patient to a nursing home. This decision was not made lightly; the physician felt he had no alternative. Nevertheless, the fact remained that Mr. S. was being sent to a nursing home to die.

Fortunately, this plan was thwarted by a psychiatrist, who correctly identified the patient's condition as tardive dyskinesia (oral buccal type), secondary to the chronic use of Stelazine. Apparently, Mr. S. had been on Stelazine, 2 mg twice a day, for moderately severe anxiety for four years prior to his hospitalization, but had failed to report this to his physicians. Once this was established, Haldol was prescribed, and the dyskinesia lessened, the patient was able to swallow, and his weight loss was reversed.

Fear and lack of knowledge of psychotropic drugs, in general, and their use in medical illness, in particular, have too long prevented their sufficient and appropriate use in the control and management of the behavior of the hospitalized patient. It is my belief that these psychopharmacological agents will ultimately make the life of the patient, the physician, and the staff more tolerable under the multiple stresses of illnesses and hospitalization.

REFERENCES

1. Glassman AH: Personal communication
1a. Glassman AH, Perel JM: Plasma levels and tricyclic antidepressants. Clin Pharmacol Ther 16:198–200, 1974
2. Prange AJ Jr: Therapeutic and theoretical implications of imipramine-hormone interactions in depressive disorders. In Psychiatry (Part II), ICS 274, Proceedings of the V World Congress of Psychiatry, Mexico DF, Nov 25–Dec 4, 1971. Amsterdam, Excerpta Medica, pp. 1023–1031
3. Greenblatt DJ, Shader RI, Koch-Weser JM: Slow absorption of intramuscular chloridiazepoxide. New Engl J Med 29:1116–1118, 1974
4. Hillestead L, Hansen T, Melsom N, Drivenes A: Diazepam metabolism in normal man, parts I and II. Clin Pharmacol Ther 16:479–489, 1974
5. Bidder TG: Personal communication
6. Greenblatt OJ, Shader RI: The clinical choice of sedative-hypnotics. Ann Intern Med 77:99–100, 1972
7. Fann WE, Schmidt D, Oates JA: The effect of antacids on the blood levels of chlopromazines. Clin Pharmacol Ther 14:135, 1973
8. Fann WE, Janowsky DS, Davis JM, Oates JA: Chlorpromazine reversal of the antihypertensive action of guanethidine. Lancet 2:436–437, 1971
9. Davis JM, Bartlett E, Termini BA: Overdosage of psychotropic drugs: a review. Dis Nerv Syst 22:157–164, 246–256, March and April, 1968
10. Schiff L (ed): Disease of the Liver, 3rd ed. Philadelphia, Lippincott, 1969, pp. 392–394, 560–565

BIBLIOGRAPHY

Bennett W, Singer I, Coggins C: A practical guide to drug usage in adult patients with impaired renal function. JAMA 214(8):1468, 1970

Davidson JRT, Raft D, Lewis BF, Gebhardt: Psychotropic drugs in general medical and surgical wards of a teaching hospital. Arch Gen Psychiatry 32:507–511, 1975

Goodman L, Gilman A: The Pharmacological Basis of Therapeutics, 5th ed. New York, Macmillan, 1974

Greenblatt DJ, Shader RI, Koch-Weser JM: Psychotropic drug use in the Boston area. Arch Gen Psychiatry 32:518–521, 1975

Hollister L: Adverse reactions to phenothiazines. JAMA 189:311–313, 1964

Klein D, Davis J: Diagnosis and Drug Treatment of Psychiatric Disorders. Baltimore, Williams & Wilkins, 1969

Shader RI, Di Mascia I, Appleton WS: Psychotropic Drug Side-Effects: Clinical and Theoretical Perspectives. Baltimore: Williams & Wilkins, 1970

Chapter 10

The Surgical Patient

Francis D. Baudry and Alfred Wiener

INTRODUCTION

A chamber of horrors, calculated to arouse the most severe anxieties, would certainly include:

1. Fear of death or mutilation or pain.
2. Uncertainty about the future.
3. Feelings of helplessness and isolation.
4. Anxiety provoked by a strange environment.
5. Relatively impersonal and unresponsive caretakers.
6. Violation of privacy; constant intrusion into the core of one's existence—the body.

Such is the setting of the contemporary surgical service as seen by the patient.

All of the above-mentioned stresses are potentially pathogenic. The point is made throughout this book that the degree of trauma they confer on the patient will depend in part on the particular individual's customary modes of adaptation and his ability to cope with stress. It will also depend on the efforts of the surgical staff. If the patient has been adequately prepared for his ordeal, instead of being overwhelmed by fears of the unknown, he will be able to remind himself that this is what the doctor told him would happen. The fundamental assumption is that, by and large, appropriate knowledge of a stressful situation fosters adaptation, while ignorance impedes it. Moreover, the fact that the patient may not want to be told what he must expect should not deter the physician from proceeding tactfully. Inadequate preparation often gives rise to resentment and may heighten anxiety, both prior to and after the procedure.

The prospect of surgery will normally evoke anxiety. (In fact, the absence of anxiety under such circumstances may be pathogenic.) The most common defense mechanism encountered is denial, varying from partial to global. Other mechanisms come into play as well. These include regression to a more childlike attitude, with passive surrender and overidealization of the hospital and the surgeon.

More obsessional patients will rely on a process of intellectualization and identification with the surgeon (seen in the patient who reads a great deal about his illness and knows the statistics). In patients who do not feel equal to the task of coping with the surgical stress, feelings of hopelessness and helplessness may be a prelude to depressive reactions. In patients who, by nature, are suspicious of others, a paranoid attitude may become more evident.

The realistic threat of mutilation is particularly likely to trigger unresolved castration anxiety. Clinically, one may see a derivative of this anxiety, for example, multiple somatic complaints and undue fearfulness about any activity, or a defense against this anxiety, which may take the form of verbal denial or denial in action, as exemplified by the patient who is boisterous, flirts with the nurses, masturbates openly, or exercises inappropriately after a coronary. These manifestations are fed by other anxieties and may have other meanings, but in general they represent an attempt by the patient to deal with his fear of bodily damage.

Anxieties surrounding the issue of death (and separation) take so many different forms that we will mention only the more obvious manifestations: depression, an inability to be alone, and an endless seeking of reassurance. If the patient uses denial to defend against his fear of death, he may appear excessively jovial before an operation. The anticipation of anesthesia, in particular, is likely to arouse anxieties about death, not waking up, passivity, mutilation, rape, and uncontrolled behavior during anesthesia.

> The psychiatrist was asked to see a 43-year-old woman who required a hysterectomy for fibroids and refused to sign her operative consent form. He discovered that she was afraid she might "talk" during anesthesia and discuss the extramarital affairs she felt was responsible for her fibroids. (She saw the surgery as her punishment.) On reassurance that she would not divulge such information during anesthesia, she readily agreed to the operation and had an uneventful postoperative course.

A patient's fear of uncontrolled behavior while under general anesthesia is an important consideration in cases where it is possible to use a spinal anesthetic.

Conflicts around helplessness and passivity may take various forms. The patient may become *too* passive and react via withdrawal and excessive regression—refusing to feed or care for himself. Or the patient may be unable to tolerate passivity—bed rest, diet, inaction. Another patient may rebel noisily against the hospital routine. Because of the anxiety of the surgical staff over his disruptive behavior, this patient is more likely to be referred for psychiatric evaluation than is the overly passive patient.

Pain or its anticipation is a common stress that usually becomes an issue in the postoperative period. Pain may be intensified as a response to the threat of body mutilation, separation, and narcissistic concern about bodily integrity. An ability to tolerate pain is associated with trust in one's caretakers and optimism about the outcome of illness.

However, just as some patients complain of pain constantly, others tolerate too much pain. The stoic patient believes that an inability to tolerate pain is a sign of weakness, and refrains from asking for analgesics even when such requests would be justified.

The Treatment Setting

The main actor of the drama, the surgeon, who spends most of his time in the operating room, is hardly ever seen on the ward. Contact with the patient is limited to brief morning and evening visits. Given his busy schedule, he has time to deal only with the essentials—wound healing, infections, intake-output, and major complications. Only bizarre manifestations of psychological states gain his attention. Even then, he may not have the time, knowledge, or motivation to deal with the patient's psychological needs.

Perhaps by far the greatest problem is a breakdown in communication at all levels, not only between patient and surgeon, but also among members of the professional staff. This is especially apparent in complicated cases, such as open heart surgery, where many different services and teams are involved, each one concerned with a small aspect of the patient's care. In such cases, the patient may receive scattered bits of information, with no one person assuming responsibility for presenting the total situation. In this context, the patient's main psychological caretakers will be the nurses and nurse's aides. With the growing trend toward primary care, the nurse somewhat reluctantly finds herself in the front lines. She bears the brunt of the patient's emotional upheavals; but, like the surgeon, her capacities to deal with psychological distress of any kind are limited.

The strain and hardship on the nursing staff working on a surgical service must not be underestimated. The nurses on our peripheral vascular service are expected to provide psychological support for the elderly and diabetic patients, who are faced with the prospect of increasingly severe and mutilating operations, often only palliative in nature and accompanied by much suffering, depression, and hopelessness. Some nurses become quite despondent in this setting; others begin to experience frightening nightmares, and, as a way of protecting themselves, isolate themselves from the patients' suffering.

Because the nurse spends the most time with the patient, and because the surgeon is relatively absent from the postoperative scene, the nurse will be the one to recognize emotional complications. Unfortunately, however, at Montefiore she is not free to request assistance in managing the patient. She must first speak with the surgeon, who, for a variety of reasons, rarely acquiesces to her request for consultation. In some instances, the surgeon is essentially unfamiliar with the function of the psychiatrist; consequently, he is afraid that the psychiatrist may do damage to his patient. He may be afraid that his own inadequacies, that is, his indifference to his patient's psychological well-being, will be exposed. Another obstacle is his narcissism: the surgeon may feel he should be able to manage his patient's emotional reaction himself.

Recently, partly in response to the demands of patients and their families, some hospital administrations have altered their neutralist stance and have installed patient advocates on a number of surgical wards. The job of these patient advocates is to act as intermediaries between the forgotten person—the patient—and an increasingly harassed surgical team.

PSYCHOLOGICAL TASKS ON THE SURGICAL SERVICE

Patient Evaluation

Patient evaluation begins with a routine history taking, which may point up certain problems:

History of previous surgical experience. The patient should be asked about his previous psychological reactions to anesthesia and about any complications that may have occurred in connection with past surgery, such as an unduly protracted hospital stay. In addition, he should be asked which aspects of his earlier surgical experience were most unpleasant, or difficult, or most frightening for him.

Details of surgical experience of relatives and close friends. It is important to obtain information about the surgical experience of family members and close friends because some patients believe that they are sure to suffer the same fate as that of a close relative or friend, especially if that fate was unfortunate. As a result, their fears of a contemplated surgical procedure may greatly exceed the actual risk involved.

The patient's perception and anticipated outcome of his illness. The patient's concept of what is wrong with him, and why, may reveal distortions in his thinking about his illness and his body. The patient should also be encouraged to verbalize his thoughts and fantasies concerning the effects of the operation, how long it will take him to recover, and the extent to which he feels his life will change as a result of surgery.

> The psychiatrist was called in to see a panic-stricken woman awaiting a mastectomy for carcinoma of the breast. Much to his surprise, her main concern was the fear that her breathing would be permanently impaired postoperatively, for she believed that her breasts were an essential organ of respiration. Clarification of the physiological reality by the psychiatrist helped to allay her anxiety.

"Spotting" Patients Who Are Likely to Develop Emotional Complications

The surgeon should attempt to identify patients who present a psychological risk both preoperatively and postoperatively. The following patients are most likely to develop emotional complications:

Patients with a previous history of psychotic decompensation of psychiatric consultation. The routine history taking should include questions concerning previous psychiatric illness or hospitalization. Patients with such a history are likely candidates for psychiatric decompensation under the stress of the surgical experience.

> A 32-year-old woman was carefully evaluated physiologically for mitral surgery; preoperative studies included catheterization and pulmonary function tests. Ten days postoperatively the nurse noted the onset of insomnia and irritability; the next night the patient refused to go to her room because "it was gassed." She was reassured by the nurse and seen the following morning by a cardiologist, whose chart note stated, "There is a need for a psychiatric consultation at this time." Twelve hours later the patient became overtly psychotic, that is, she hallucinated and displayed overt paranoid delusions. She was then seen by a psychiatric consultant and eventually transferred to the psychiatric service, where she made an uneventful recovery in approximately two weeks. During her stay on the psychiatric service, information was elicited from her

husband to the effect that the patient had had a brief acute psychotic episode during another hospitalization six months previously.

Clearly, if the patient's total history had been elicited in advance, proper precautions could have been taken—such as inquiry into the patient's particular fears—and specific reassurance could have been given. In addition, recognition of the early signs of the patient's postoperative delirium (insomnia, irritability, and her conviction that the room was gassed) would have allowed earlier treatment with tranquilizers, avoiding the fulminating psychosis and the extra stress on the patient's heart, which had just been operated on.

Patients who refuse to undergo indicated surgery, either by threatening to sign out of the hospital, or by refusing to sign a consent form. The surgeon must be aware that the uncooperative and negative attitude of the patient who threatens to sign out of the hospital, or refuses to sign a consent form, is, in fact, evidence of severe anxiety or even panic.

> A man in his sixties, who was admitted to the hospital for an elective herniorraphy, developed an upper respiratory infection during the preoperative work-up, necessitating postponement of the operation. He became angry and suspicious, blamed the doctors for his setback, and insisted that if he had been a private patient this would never have happened. He then threatened to sign out of the hospital.
> When a member of the staff talked with him, it became apparent that the patient did not expect to survive the operation, and had dealt with his resultant near panic with anger and accusatory behavior. This house doctor expressed his interest and concern for the patient by visiting him daily, even on his day off. The patient, in turn, developed a strong and trusting childlike attachment to the doctor, kissing his hand and weeping with tears of gratitude whenever he saw him. He underwent surgery performed by this doctor, and made a successful recovery.

Patients whose relationships with the staff are deteriorating. Many patients make unreasonable demands on the staff, or relate to them in a cantankerous, complaining, and accusatory manner. Others refuse to comply with routine hospital procedures, or do so only under pressure. Whenever the staff–patient relationship becomes inordinately difficult, emotional problems within the patient may be the cause of the friction.

Such patients are often unable to express their feelings in words, or may even be totally unaware of their feelings. They can only communicate with the staff through their behavior. The difficulty in dealing with them stems in part from the almost universal reaction of anger elicited in the staff by their disruptive actions. The staff feel that the patient is challenging their professional competence; they perceive him as "ungrateful" and are angry because he interferes with the care of patients who are "really sick." The essential message the patient is trying to convey is lost.

Patients with unrealistic or magical expectations concerning their operation. Patients with unrealistic or magical expectations should not be permitted to undergo surgery until they have been made aware of what they can reasonably expect from the surgical procedure. Such an approach spares the patient and the surgeon much subsequent disillusionment and postoperative difficulty. Many patients requesting plastic surgery fall into this category, especially if the defect to be corrected is relatively minor. Teen-agers or young adults who blame their social failures on some minor facial defect or breast abnormality as a way of not facing major personality liabilities should not be operated on. Unrealistic or magical expectations are also prominent in patients with chronic disease, for example, a patient whose chronic heart ailment has made him an invalid may expect to be completely cured by surgery. The more unrealistic the patient's expectations are, the stronger the possibility that he will develop adverse emotional reactions to his illness in the future, unless appropriate prophylactic measures are taken.

Patients who present special diagnostic problems and in whom the need for an operation is uncertain. The surgeon must be able to evaluate the meaning of the patient's complaint. Patients do not always present symptoms or complaints to get relief. In presenting their symptoms they may be expressing a demand for care or reproach, an appeal, or displaced anxiety or depression; a patient may even offer a symptom defensively, that is, to hide another symptom he is too frightened to bring up. Unless the surgeon understands what is troubling the patient, he cannot deal effectively with the symptom. This is, of course, a truism in clinical medicine, but it is often overlooked when an organic explanation for the patient's symptom is available. It has been our experience that even when a surgeon recognizes a clear-cut emotional problem, he often handles it with blanket reassurance and drugs; rarely does he attempt to analyze the situation and to take appropriate measures.

Much unnecessary surgery is performed because the surgeon accepts the patient's surface complaint at face value, instead of evaluating it in the context of the patient's personality and current life situation. The patient who consciously or unconsciously seeks an operation as a temporary way out of a difficult situation is a common phenomenon.

The less certain the surgeon is of the need to operate, the stronger the imperative for the patient to be evaluated psychologically. Difficult diagnostic problems such as vague complaints of abdominal pain, or pelvic complaints of obscure etiology in women, are classical examples of such dilemmas.

Patients who show too much or too little concern in the preoperative period. As noted above, some preoperative anxiety is normal. When anxiety is blatantly absent, or when the patient appears overenthusiastic about the operation, demands it even before it is offered, or in any way manifests lack of appropriate emotional responses at any level, the possibility that postoperative complications and even unexplained deaths may occur is heightened.

Among patients who show a pathological lack of concern about surgery, we would include persons who, consciously or unconsciously, expect to die, whether they verbalize this or not. Intuitively, or at the cost of bitter experience, many surgeons have adopted the practice of rejecting such patients for surgery, provided they are identified in time. It is common knowledge that such patients have the remarkable capacity of accomplishing their death wish, even when the "operation is a success."

Kennedy and Bakst,[1] who studied the impact of emotional factors on the outcome of cardiac surgery at Montefiore Hospital, found that a high level of preoperative anxiety, when combined with poor motivation, led to a high postoperative mortality rate in open heart surgery cases. This finding has important practical implications: Kennedy and Bakst suggest that these risk factors should be identified and worked with prior to surgery. Moreover, if, despite psychiatric intervention, a high level of anxiety persists, surgery may be contraindicated if it is not immediately essential for the preservation of life.

Kimball,[2] who also attempted to correlate the level of anxiety with the postcardiac surgery death rate, came up with the same results: more anxious patients had a higher death rate. However, Kimball did not control for the fact that sicker patients may be more anxious secondary to their illness. It was not clear, therefore, whether the high level of anxiety was primarily a psychosomatic or a somatopsychic event.

Cassem and Hackett[3] found that the outcome of surgery was greatly affected by the preoperative expectation. For example, patients who had a pessimistic outlook had a pessimistic outcome.

In fact, evaluating the patient's preoperative status and predicting outcome can be problematic. Kilpatrick and his co-workers,[4] who used psychological test data to predict the outcome of open heart surgery, were able to correctly classify survivors and fatalities. However, the guidelines noted above need to be tempered by a clinical assessment of the patient's total personality and adaptive strengths. Words or expressions out of context may be misleading and may foster an unwarranted judgment that surgery is contraindicated on psychological grounds.

> Mr. S., a 53-year-old clothier, with longstanding rheumatic heart disease and valvular damage, had become progressively disabled, and was finally unable to work. While he was awaiting surgery, his carefully compensated cardiac status of some twenty years finally gave way, and he verbalized many pessimistic, anxiety-laden, and grandiose thoughts that made his surgeon sufficiently uncertain of the outcome of surgery to request a psychiatric evaluation. For example, Mr. S. said, "I'll never get off the table; the surgeon plans to draw and quarter me like a chicken. If I do get off the table, no woman will be safe; and I'll be so strong, no man will be safe from my anger."

Since Mr. S. was not in imminent danger from his heart disease, the surgeon felt that surgery should be postponed until a psychiatric evaluation was made. The psychiatrist learned that the patient was sad and worried, but that he looked forward hopefully to the operation, and was optimistic about its outcome. Despite his anxiety-laden and pessimistic statements, Mr. S. was not particularly depressed, and the content of his fears was seen as the expression of moderately severe anxiety, in keeping with his prior hypochondriacal brooding. But they were in no way suggestive of a "death wish."

An important clue to the patient's real lack of anxiety and pessimism was his wish not to discuss his worries, coupled with the statement that he was content to "Let the doctor worry; he knows best." The surgeon then performed the operation, and one day postoperative, Mr. S., attached to various kinds of apparatus and confined to his bed, said he finally felt he could relax with all the lights, equipment, and people looking after him.

PREOPERATIVE AND POSTOPERATIVE PSYCHOLOGICAL INTERVENTION

Preoperative Psychological Preparation

The surgeon is the person best qualified to prepare the patient for surgery. He is the most informed and, from the patient's point of view, the most threatening—and, therefore, potentially the most reassuring. However, in practice (often by default), the task of preparation is left to others, or even entirely ignored. The person next best suited for the task is the family doctor (if there is one). Occasionally, in especially difficult cases, the psychiatrist may have to be involved.

The time required to properly prepare a patient is a function of the complexity of the hospitalization, the patient's past surgical history, the degree of postoperative mutilation that is anticipated, the overt anxiety of the patient, and, finally, the patient's capacity to assimilate what he is told.

One or two preparatory "sessions" will suffice in less complicated situations. In certain types of operations where the diagnosis is uncertain, such as breast biopsy, the main anxiety is related to the uncertainty of the diagnosis. This can only be resolved by the operation, and any delay for whatever reason allows the build up of fear, which no amount of preparation can alleviate. In contrast to these situations, delay is advantageous in preoperative conditions such as cardiac surgery, for example, in which there is a high degree of anxiety based on many intrapsychic factors that can be identified and ameliorated prior to surgery to reduce the risk of morbidity and mortality.

First and foremost, the doctor must tell the patient what is in store for him, specifically, what sensory experiences he will undergo (what he will see, feel, or hear); what he may see when he awakens from the operation, especially if he is to spend some time in the recovery room; and so forth. Hopefully, in the course of providing such factual information, the doctor will not only be able to correct the patient's misconceptions and distortions, but will also be able to dispel fantasies surrounding the surgical procedure.

In a classical work on surgical stress, Janis[5] alludes to the "work of worrying": in order to better prepare oneself for unpleasant experiences, it is necessary to go through the work of worrying (as an analogy to the work of mourning). As with the process of inoculation, it becomes beneficial to stimulate anxiety in small management doses in order to spare the patient greater anxiety. Specifically, the patient must be persuaded to confront emotionally certain of the realistic aspects of the surgical experience ahead of time so that he can assimilate them.

Availability of the doctor and his clarification of the situation are the best antidotes to fears mobilized by a real danger. This serves to cement the doctor–patient relationship, to show the patient that the doctor cares about him and his plight, and that he is ready to help him through his ordeal. A good doctor–patient relationship makes it possible for the patient to voice his fears. The usefulness of this verbalization has been demonstrated repeatedly.

The patient's questions should be answered with a view toward fostering trust in his surgeon and encouraging realistic planning. However, it is important not to reassure the patient at first, although this might seem tempting. Reassurance that comes too soon or that is excessive is likely to make the patient more anxious or to give him the feeling that the doctor hasn't been listening to him or that he doesn't know what he is talking about. It is one of the basic tenets of preoperative preparation that the doctor must elicit the patient's misconceptions and fantasies before he can provide appropriate reassurance and information in accordance with the patient's psychological needs.

Finally, certain types of situations are almost always fraught with emotional complications, and the preparation of these patients requires special care and sensitivity. These include mutilating operations, such as mastectomies, amputations, colostomies, operations on the heart and brain, and hysterectomies.

Postoperative Psychological Problems and Their Management

Certain psychological dysfunctions may become manifest during the postoperative period.

Delirium. The emergence of an acute organic brain syndrome is extremely common in some surgical procedures, for example, cardiac surgery, prostate operation in the elderly, and surgery in patients who are already organically impaired. The manifestations are often transient, may only occur at night, and are frequently missed by the staff. They include irritability, confusion, disorientation, and illusions, which may progress to active delusions of a persecutory nature.

The elderly patient, because of his already compromised brain functioning, is especially prone to preoperative and postoperative psychological complications. The unfamiliar hospital environment may produce catastrophic-like reactions preoperatively; postoperatively delirium is frequently seen following the use of general anesthesia.

Excessive anxiety. This may be manifested by irritability, insomnia, excessive need for pain medication, and various somatic disturbances, such as hyperventilation, tachycardia, and arrythmias. In addition, the patient's characteristic method of coping with anxiety will become exaggerated and may lead to management problems, for example, increased obsessionality, with a need to control, and counterphobic behavior. Blanket reassurance is usually useless; effective therapeutic intervention consists of eliciting the source of the patient's anxiety. For example, he may be literally afraid to move at all, or even to breathe for fear that his body will break open. Once the specific source or sources of the patient's anxiety have been identified, a rational therapeutic approach becomes apparent.

Excessive pain, with increased demands for narcotics. The problem of pain is complicated and is discussed in detail in Chapter 8. Suffice it to say here that emotional factors enter into the postoperative manifestations of pain to a far greater extent than is realized; that many patients receive inadequate postoperative analgesia; and that pain is often a somatic communication of emotional distress. The psychiatrist can facilitate the interpretation of this latent message.

Depression. Depression may be manifested by insomnia, anorexia, noncooperation (e.g., refusing to walk or to cough), feelings of hopelessness, apathy, and so on. Withdrawal and regression, as a result of severe depressive reactions, may require electroshock therapy as a life-saving measure.

Following surgery, withdrawal and severe regression may be seen in infantile personalities. The patient may lie motionless, refusing to care for his basic needs—feeding, elimination, and so forth. The management of such patients is difficult and time-consuming, and may require a total push approach involving physicians, nurses, family, psychiatrists, and others.

In treating postoperative depression, supportive psychological care, including ventilation of anxieties, reassurance, reality testing, and promoting the reevaluation of the postsurgical self, that is, mourning for the lost body parts or functions, is essential. (The information in Chap. 3 about the psychological management of the medically ill applies here.) In addition, psychopharmacological agents to allay excessive anxiety and sufficient analgesics to minimize pain should be employed.

The Function of the Psychiatrist

The psychiatrist has multiple possibilities of being of service on a surgical ward. In addition to seeing specific patients in his capacity as a consultant, he may also spot patients who are in great need of help but who for one reason or another have not been identified. Particularly on a surgical service, only a very small number of patients who could benefit from a psychiatric consultation are actually identified. Another, and perhaps even more crucial, function of the psychiatrist is to identify patients for whom surgery is not appropriate. This would include patients with hypochondriasis, conversion reactions, depressive reactions, psychotic delusions, and the malingerers—all of whom may present with complaints that are actually psychogenic. It is the psychiatrist's task to persuade the surgeon of the need to properly evaluate the patient's demands for surgical intervention—no matter how urgent these demands may be.

Finally, the psychiatrist is often called upon to perform a "clearance" function. For example, he may be asked to assess the mental functioning in patients who refuse surgery despite the urgency of a procedure, or to evaluate the ability of a particular patient to deal with the psychological stresses of multiple, disabling surgical procedures.

At times, the surgeon may attempt to abdicate his responsibility to decide to operate when the indications for surgery are ambiguous, and the possible gains of intervention minimal. Patients with organic disease who use illness and incapacity as a protection against being functional and self-sustaining are the most difficult to evaluate. Such patients often request surgery with an intensity that makes the surgeon uncomfortable. The surgeon may then try to place the burden of decision making onto the psychiatrist, with one of the following typical requests: "Evaluate patient's depression or functional overlay," or "The patient's complaints seem out of keeping with her disability; please advise as to whether she will benefit from surgery." Such requests for psychiatric clearance must be evaluated carefully if the psychiatrist is not to be seduced into making a decision for the surgeon.

> Mr. Q., a 46-year-old accountant, had fallen at work ten years prior to his current hospitalization. He had sought no medical treatment for two months following his accident at which time the pain had become unbearable. A medical consultation revealed a fracture and skin ulceration, and a series of operations was performed to correct the chronic osteomyelitis, which the surgeons felt could lead eventually to bone tumor requiring amputation. Thirteen previous plastic surgical procedures had failed, in all likelihood because of the patient's unconscious need to undo the result by constantly picking at the graft.
>
> Mr. Q. desperately wanted his surgeon to make one last try, using a new method that would allow a flap from his chest to be grafted onto the anterior lower leg. This would require that he maintain an almost impossible position for several weeks while the graft took.

Ostensibly, the surgeon wanted the psychiatrist to decide whether the patient was psychologically eligible for surgery in view of his history. However, it became clear in the course of a combined clinical conference that the psychiatrist was being asked, inappropriately, to make the decision for or against surgery. Once he had made the limits of his responsibility clear, the psychiatrist was able to realistically offer a variety of psychological interventions that could assist the patient preoperatively and postoperatively if the surgeon so desired. The patient's motivation, capacity to tolerate pain and discomfort, and his plea that he be given this last chance to save his leg all argued in his favor. And, in fact, these strengths sustained the patient through an exceedingly difficult, but ultimately successful, fourteenth operative procedure.

It should be obvious that in order to be most helpful, the psychiatrist must be clearly informed of the exact nature of the problem confronting the surgeon, and of the questions in the surgeon's mind—questions that up to the time of the psychiatric consultation may have only been vaguely formulated. Often, the psychiatrist must spend time with the nurses, house staff, and surgeons in order to evaluate subtle factors in their personal interaction that may have contributed to the present problem. There is no place here for jargon or evasion on the part of the psychiatrist; on the other hand, if the surgeon is to benefit from the psychiatrist's expertise, he must be willing to spend sufficient time with the psychiatrist to permit him to get an accurate picture of intrastaff and staff–patient relationships on the ward.

In a sense, the surgical service of a general hospital simulates a laboratory situation. It offers the psychiatrist a unique opportunity to witness, at first hand, the nature and effects of acute stress not only on patients but on word personnel. In addition, the psychiatrist has an invaluable exposure to the whole array of coping mechanisms available to patients. Thus, the psychiatrist comes to realize that most patients are able to surmount what may appear to be insurmountable stress, with relative impunity. Psychiatrists are so adept at spotting psychopathology that they forget, or don't have the experience, to evaluate the coping mechanisms that most individuals are able to bring to stressful situations. The surgical ward provides an ideal setting for any research endeavor in the study of both physiological and psychological parameters of stress.

Finally, psychiatrists do not have their diagnoses and interventions tested by post-mortem examinations. However, on an acute surgical ward the liaison psychiatrist's opinions are open to challenge. Any preoperative recommendation or treatment plan is tested on the spot, and the outcome of the recommendations can be assessed quickly. This can be a sobering, if not chastizing, experience. Most important, it can be an invaluable learning experience.

REFERENCES

1. Kennedy J, Bakst H: The influence of emotions on the outcome of cardiac surgery: a predictive study. Bull NY Acad Med 42:811, 1966
2. Kimball CP: Psychological response to the experience of open heart surgery, I. Am J Psychiatry 126:3, September 1969
3. Cassem N, Hackett TP: Psychiatric consultation in a coronary care unit. Ann Intern Med 75:9–14, 1971
4. Kilpatrick DG, Miller WC, Allain AN, Huggins MB, Lee WH Jr: The use of psychological test data to predict open-heart surgery outcome: a prospective study. Psychosom Med 37(1):62–73, 1975
5. Janis IL: Psychological Stress: Psychoanalytic and Behavioral Studies of Surgical Patients. New York, Wiley, 1958

BIBLIOGRAPHY

Baudry F, Wiener A, Hurwitt ES: Indications for psychiatric consultations on a surgical service. Surgery 60:993, 1966

Bergmann T, Freud A: Children in Hospital. New York, International Universities Press, 1965

Stehlin J, Beach K: Enlisting relatives in cancer management. Med World News 8:112, 1967

Chapter 11

The Physician's Response to the Dying Patient

James Spikes and Jimmie Holland

The psychology of the dying patient has been explored extensively in recent literature,[1-7] with the result that an impressive body of knowledge now exists to aid the primary physician in his work with these patients. However, the implementation of this knowledge has been minimal at best. Nor can we expect these or future studies in this area to produce major improvements in medical care. For the physician cannot be expected to assimilate the data (and the recommendations they incorporate) unless he has been able to deal with the stresses such patients typically evoke. The liaison psychiatrist is ideally suited, by virtue of his relationship to the ward staff, to deal with these psychological issues.

Caring for the dying patient may elicit significant stress in the physician who has not resolved his unconscious feelings of omnipotence.[4, 8-11] These feelings may find expression in his image of himself as the powerful healer, as indestructible, and/or as a destructive force. And each of these unconscious attitudes may, in turn, have adverse effects on his ability to provide optimal care for the patient.*

They may, for example, color the physician's reaction to the intense,

---

* Two concepts implicit in this chapter are subject to possible misunderstanding and should, therefore, be clarified at the outset. First, although the data presented derive from our experience on the oncology service, the attitudes discussed may be encountered among physicians faced with the problem of caring for the dying patient, regardless of the nature of the patient's disease or the clinical setting in which he is seen. Second, it would be erroneous for physicians and patients to automatically equate cancer with death; many forms of malignancy are now amenable to treatment.

anxious patient who bombards him with such questions as: "How long do I have to live?" It has been our experience that many physicians respond to such questions with false reassurance or avoidance; others give the patient or family member a definite answer to the question, when, in fact, it is impossible to predict the temporal outcome of the patient's illness. Little consideration is given to what this question might mean to the particular person who is asking it, and often no attempt is made to understand its meaning.

Closer examination of this kind of response reveals that it represents an attempt on the part of the physician to ward off his own disappointment with his professional fallibility. He is not sure he will be able to cure the illness; nor can he even predict its course or outcome. It is easier, therefore, to dispose of his anxiety by giving a definite answer where none is possible, or by avoiding the patient. Exposure and clarification of these unconscious attitudes by the liaison psychiatrist will foster an easier and more productive interaction between members of the medical staff and their dying patients.[11] Unfortunately, because these attitudes are so firmly entrenched, attempts at exposure often lead to extreme anxiety and defensiveness on the part of the medical staff, thereby creating potentially destructive tensions between them and the psychiatrist. Therefore, the purpose of this chapter is not only to describe these unconscious attitudes and their consequences, but to elucidate the problems of the psychiatrist as he attempts to deal with them.

UNCONSCIOUS FANTASIES OF OMNIPOTENCE

The Powerful Healer

The most troublesome responses to dying patients stem from the physician's unconscious need to preserve his image as a "powerful healer." If this attitude, which is also the most pervasive, is not brought to light and dealt with, the doctor experiences a feeling of personal failure. He may feel frustrated, hopeless, helpless, and angry, and then employ certain maladaptive measures to deal with these feelings. The following extract from a weekly liaison meeting with house officers on the oncology ward illustrates repercussions of this attitude.

> A young woman intern was taking care of a 42-year-old woman who had metastatic carcinoma of the breast. In discussing her patient, she said, "I feel there is nothing I can do for the patient. No matter what I do, she is still going to die, and that means I have failed. I get out of her room as fast as I can because I don't want

to think about her. I really get depressed when I come here in the morning."

Further examination of this situation by the group revealed that there were many things that this doctor had already done and could still do for this patient. Her pain could be controlled, and an uncomfortable pleural effusion could be tapped. But, more important, the doctor could help this patient and her family to explore their feelings about her illness. The intern and the other house doctors were then able to see that her feelings of despair were the result of her need to succeed by saving the patient from death. If she could not offer the patient a cure, she had nothing to offer. Consequently, she was unable to realistically evaluate her capacities to care for the patient.

The fact that patients and families also view the physician as a powerful healer compounds his problem. If he is unable to achieve a cure, the patient and family may feel that he has failed them. If the physician agrees with them, he may seek to ward off feelings of guilt and depression by defensive reactions of anger or avoidance.

A 65-year-old man was admitted to the oncology service with a diagnosis of metastatic carcinoma of the prostate. His wife felt extremely guilty about his condition, and continually reproached herself for not having urged the patient earlier to consult a physician. One of the ways she was able to handle this feeling was to blame her husband's doctors for not beginning treatment soon enough, and for not being more diligent in their care.

One day she attended a family conference in which the psychological care of terminal patients was being discussed. After listening quietly for a few minutes, she suddenly exploded, "How can you doctors just sit around here talking? Why aren't you in the laboratory trying to find a cure for this disease?" Immediately, one of the doctors replied, "I never heard anything so awful! You have absolutely no respect! How dare you talk to us that way!"

The doctor had clearly reacted defensively—that is, as if this criticism had some basis in truth against which he had to defend himself. If this sense of guilt, which stemmed from his anger at the patient—and at himself, because of his helplessness—had not been operative, he would have been able, as he subsequently was, to explore the meaning of the outburst. The doctor's anger and the anger the patient's wife felt served the same purpose. In both instances, it was a desperate attempt to ward off feelings that they had failed the patient.

Another reaction to the frustration of the physician's image of himself as the powerful healer is the emergence of wishes that the patient would die.

These wishes can occur as isolated thoughts or as preoccupations that take on a ruminative quality. In either form, such reactions are natural, and one often sees them in families of patients, especially of patients who are exposed to extreme suffering. These wishes become troublesome to a physician when he recognizes that they are related not to feelings of empathy for the dying patient, but to feelings of anger toward him. In that event, they give rise to feelings of guilt and self-reproach. When they are examined more closely, it seems clear that such death wishes toward the patient stem from the fact that the physician sees the patient as a constant reminder of his own "inadequacy." If he did not have to confront the patient each day, he could continue to view himself as a "powerful healer." Instead of turning his anger inward, which would result in depression, the physician has the troublesome wish that the patient would die.

A third common reaction to frustration of the doctor's self-image is overtreatment of the patient. The patient may realize that his body cannot hold out any longer and be ready to die. Sometimes the physician's reaction at this point is to intensify therapy, even in ways that can make the patient (and his family) more uncomfortable. Moreover, the physician may even become angry with the patient who refuses further therapy and openly expresses the wish to be left alone to die. The physician is plagued with thoughts that he has not done enough for the patient, or that he did not start appropriate treatment at the optimal time. And there is another possibility: in an attempt to ward off these feelings of guilt, he may become critical of colleagues. He may attempt to "blame" the patient's deteriorating condition on others. It is as if he were saying, "It is not I who am imperfect, but you."

The Indestructible Self

An important corollary to the attitude of the "powerful healer" is the "indestructible self." Empathizing with patients who are dying necessarily evokes anxiety about one's own death. Many physicians express this anxiety by saying that they cannot talk with these patients because they "overidentify" with them. This becomes particularly apparent when the patient possesses some of the social characteristics of the physician—age, profession, or ethnic background. This anxiety is rooted in the physician's fear, and need to avoid awareness of the fact, that just as he cannot save his patient's life, he may not be able to save his own. As a result of this anxiety, he often avoids the patient, becomes irritated with him, or falsely reassures him.

A young resident on the oncology ward who was taking care of a young dental student with advanced lymphosarcoma reported that his patient tried to engage him in conversation each morning on rounds. The patient would express concern about his condition; the resident would tell him not to worry and leave the room. The resident felt uncomfortable about this, realizing that the patient might benefit from talking with him, if only for a few minutes. When his thoughts were explored further, it occurred to him that what he feared was that the patient might express his sadness about not being able to finish dental school, or about not being able to get married as he had planned. When we asked him how he would feel if his patient began to cry, the resident replied that he was afraid that he would break down himself. He then said that if the patient expressed his feelings it would make him aware that this could happen to him, and that he did not want to let such thoughts even cross his mind.

The Destructive Force

The attitude evoked by the physician's image of himself as a destructive force is closely related to the attitude of the powerful healer through two unconscious mechanisms: If the physician is so powerful that he can cure everyone, he must also have tremendously destructive resources at his command; and the patient's condition constantly reminds the physician of his imperfection, which excites feelings of anger in him. The image of the destructive force may have other important determinants as well, namely, the presence of unconscious, hostile (perhaps sadistic) impulses that are defended against by strong overcompensation (reaction formations).[8]

One conscious derivative of this attitude is the physician's worrisome feeling that he may harm the patient. This attitude may interfere with treatment in several clinical situations. The first is the situation in which the doctor is treating a serious illness with potent drugs or surgical procedures that have potentially dangerous consequences or side effects.

Chapter 2 provided a good illustration of the problems that can arise in this situation. While treating a young man who had leukemia with chemotherapeutic drugs, Dr. N., a young intern, was distressed by the thought that instead of helping her patient, she was "poisoning" him. She feared that she, not the illness, would cause the patient's death.

The physician's fear of hurting the patient can also lead to premature "giving up" on a patient and the consequent failure to institute or continue appropriate treatment. This can be seen particularly in the treatment of cancer when a physician may make a judgment to let his patient "die in peace," and not make available to him therapeutic procedures that may prolong life, and, in some cases, may even cure the disease. The reasons given, "I won't subject him to mutilating surgery," or "I won't allow those 'poisons' to be given to my patient. He's going to die anyway," are rationalizations. The doctor may make this determination in a patient who would choose to accept the stressful procedures if there were a possibility they would result in a remission of his illness. There are times when such a decision is correctly made; but there are also times when it is too easily made on psychological grounds relating to the physician's needs, instead of on the basis of either medical data or the patient's needs.

This attitude can also cause trouble when the physician is asked, usually by the patient, to discuss his illness with him. Many physicians are overcome by the fear that they will say or do something to upset the patient: "What if he asks me, 'Do I have cancer?' or 'How long do I have to live?' " They are afraid they will "let the cat out of the bag." In most cases, what the patient really wants is someone to listen to him, someone who can be both empathic and objective. Who, he asks himself, is better qualified than his own doctor? Yet, sometimes, to the patient's surprise, the person he attempts to talk to is nervous, even irritable, and cannot wait to get out of the room. Although such behavior by the physician may relate, in part, to his feelings of inadequacy in treating the patient's illness, it may also stem from his fear of hurting the patient by "saying or doing the wrong thing." It is almost as if the physician believes he may be as destructive to the patient as the illness. Instead of "poisoning" the patient with dangerous drugs, he will do it with words! Physicians who are so preoccupied with their own concerns may avoid the patient even when he wants to discuss something trivial or unrelated to the illness itself. As a result the patient begins to wonder what is so awful about him that his doctor cannot bear to spend any time with him.

The physician's unconscious image of himself as a destructive force may also cause him to respond inappropriately to the patient's crucial questions. Ideally, the physician's response to these questions will be predicated on his knowledge of the patient's personality and how he has responded to previous stresses. He can then gauge the amount of information he should provide and when and how it can be presented in the most humane way for each patient under his care. Moreover, irrespective of the patient's prognosis, the physician will never paint his picture as completely hopeless; and, at the same time, he will assure the patient of his continuing support.

The physician who feels uncomfortable about dealing with patients on this level may try to assuage his discomfort by lying to his patients. Regardless of the nature or projected course of a patient's illness, he is told, "You have a minor problem, but you'll soon be well again. There's nothing to worry about." Time and the progression of illness prove the physician a liar, and seeds of distrust are sown at a time when trust is vital. At the other extreme is the physician who prides himself on the fact that he tells every patient "the unvarnished truth," regardless of his personality and resources. "You have six months to live, there's nothing I can do for you" is a form of painful abandonment that confirms the worst fears of the patient who is not getting better. The "always tellers" and the "never tellers" have no place in this delicate area of the art of medicine. Both these positions reflect a lack of flexibility on the part of the physician and an inability to modify his behavior in response to the patient's needs.

In addition to the reactions evoked by the parameters of unresolved feelings of omnipotence described above, the physician may employ two defensive measures to deal with his sense of guilt and inadequacy: he may become overly attached to the patient, and/or he may project his feelings of failure onto the psychiatrist.

First, a mutual sense of attachment is bound to develop in the course of any doctor–patient relationship. Consequently, the death (or the impending death) of the patient will bring about a sense of loss (or anticipation of loss) in the physician.[12]

These feelings are perfectly natural unless they are carried to extremes because of the physician's own personal need to become emotionally overinvolved with the patient. In that event the patient becomes saddled with a burden he should not have to bear. If the patient is actively contributing to this overinvolvement (as is often the case), it is usually because he feels abandoned by family members or friends, who are finding it difficult to handle their own feelings about him and the nature of his illness. It will be difficult or impossible for the physician to remedy this situation if he has become overly involved with the patient. Because he has identified with the patient, he either will not approach the patient's family, or if he does approach them, he will convey his feelings of anger toward them for abandoning the patient, which will cause his efforts to induce them to alter their behavior to fail.

Second, the liaison psychiatrist may become the focus of the defensive measures the medical staff muster to handle their feelings of guilt or helplessness. These measures usually take two forms, and they may be seen separately or in combination. First, the staff may seek to relieve their discomfort by transferring the psychological care of the patient to the psychiatrist. Second, their feelings of guilt and helplessness may be projected onto the psychiatrist, who is then seen as the impotent or hurtful person.

Transfer of the Patient

A psychiatrist was called to see a 55-year-old man for evaluation of depression. The patient had been admitted with a severe right-sided hemiparesis and aphasia, which had occurred one month after a successful aortic valve replacement. The stroke was assumed to be due to an embolus from the new valve. In addition, a small coin lesion had recently been discovered on the patient's chest x-ray. The psychiatrist found the patient to be depressed, with suicidal ideation, and the patient's internist advanced the theory that the depression was due to the patient's concern over the proposed second operation to explore the etiology of the coin lesion. He suggested either immediate discharge or transfer to the psychiatry ward. The next day the patient was transferred to psychiatry. Two days later the patient's hemiparesis suddenly worsened, and the neurology consultant made a diagnosis of bronchogenic carcinoma, metastatic to the brain.

Projection

A liaison psychiatrist was called to see a young man with severe regional enteritis. Shortly after the initial interview with the psychiatrist, a perforation of the small bowel occurred, and the patient was rushed to the operating room. The patient's internist then loudly proclaimed that the psychiatrist's "stressful interview" had caused the perforation.

INTERVENTION

Essentially, the liaison psychiatrist's work with the medical staff who care for dying patients involves two processes: Educating the staff with regard to the psychological needs of the patient and his family, and helping the staff to identify and deal with their own attitudes toward these patients.

In our opinion, the second process, helping the staff to deal with their unconscious attitudes toward these patients is more important than the first, because unless the physician's unconscious attitudes are clarified, the psychiatrist's educative efforts will, in all probability, fall on deaf ears.[8-11]

In general, the most effective model for working with staff attitudes is the active, ongoing liaison program, as described in Chapter 14. There are three reasons for this. First, individual psychiatric consultation with a physician and a patient is usually too limited, both in time and in depth, to promote active growth and change. Second, weekly staff meetings with the psychiatrist in a medical setting permit discussion of a range of problems, and, at the same time, foster supportive relationships among staff members that make it easier for them to deal with their feelings. Third, contact with the psychiatrist and other group members over a period of time is usually essential for the development of the trust necessary to divulging one's feelings without fear of criticism.

The weekly liaison teaching conference has proven the most effective vehicle for promoting psychological growth in the staff, particularly when the conference is co-chaired by an appropriate medical authority figure, for example, a medical attending, who serves as a role model for the staff.[11]

The nature of the psychiatrist's interventions at such conferences can be summarized as follows:

1. He encourages the staff to ventilate their feelings toward particular patients under their care (e.g., feelings of inadequacy, guilt, anger), and attempts to foster awareness of the origins of these attitudes (i.e., unresolved feelings of omnipotence).
2. He employs reality testing with the staff to help to convince them that their feelings of worthlessness and despair have an irrational basis, to reduce their feelings of guilt, and to enable them to function more effectively.
3. He encourages open expression of grief about the impending or actual loss of particular patients.
4. He emphasizes the use of the team approach in the medical setting, since, if several persons are working with a patient, this decreases the possibility that one staff member will become overly burdened. However, one staff member must ultimately care for the patient, and the team must support the person who undertakes this task.
5. He encourages each staff doctor to find his own level of tolerance for dealing with these patients and the feelings they evoke, and helps him to accept this level of tolerance in himself—to view it as a human limit to his capacities, rather than as a personal inadequacy.[11]

The Psychiatrist

Renneker[13] has shown that all of the conflicts, attitudes, and reactions described above with regard to medical personnel may also be present in the psychiatrist, and may interfere with his ability to provide optimal psychological care for the dying patient and emotional support for the patient's doctor. If the psychiatrist has not been able to resolve these issues, he will experience the same inhibitions he observes in his medical colleagues, and he will be unable to empathize adequately, either with his medical colleagues or with their patients.

The psychiatrist must also be able to effectively handle the defensive operations of the medical staff when they involve him directly. As noted above, the staff may attempt to defend against their feelings of inadequacy by transferring the emotional care of the patient to the psychiatrist, or by projecting their own feelings of guilt and helplessness onto the psychiatrist. These behaviors may evoke certain maladaptive reactions in the psychiatrist that will impair his effectiveness.

These maladaptive reactions may take the form of *anger,* expressed directly and/or indirectly. The psychiatrist may openly criticize his medical colleagues for their behavior; he may cancel meetings and/or retreat from the medical setting. Or the maladaptive reactions may take the form of *unwarranted acceptance* by the psychiatrist of the unrealistic task the staff has asked of him—he may actually accept transfer of a patient, although the psychiatric staff are not equipped to handle the patient's urgent medical needs; and/or unwarranted acceptance of the medical staff's judgment that his intervention has caused an exacerbation of the patient's symptoms, in which event, he will become depressed and experience feelings of guilt and helplessness.

These two reactions may occur together in various combinations, or they may occur in sequence. For example, the psychiatrist sometimes accepts transfer of the patient, and then becomes angry with the staff, blaming them because he has taken on an inappropriate task.

Closer examination of these reactions in the psychiatrist reveals that they occur when he has not resolved his own feelings of omnipotence. Like the internist and the surgeon, the psychiatrist may have an unconscious image of himself as a "powerful healer." Feelings of inadequacy arise when this image is shattered. When the psychiatrist accepts an unwarranted transfer of the patient, he is trying to preserve this self-image: he will relieve the staff of their burden, accomplish some magical cure, and thereby gain their respect and admiration. When this fails, as it is bound to, the psychiatrist either becomes depressed (and feels guilty) or projects these feelings onto the staff and becomes angry with them.

Lipowski,[14] who has described some of the mechanisms discussed above with regard to the practice of liaison psychiatry in general, refers to the situation in which the psychiatrist is spurned, and perhaps deprecated, by his colleagues as one of "calumniatory denigration." Our observations and experiences indicate that this situation is most commonly and most intensely activated within the milieu of the dying patient. In no other setting do the patient, family, and medical staff become so angry, desperate, and despairing. The patient must cope with loss of function, disfigurement, and the threat of death. He projects his feelings of inadequacy onto his doctors, and becomes outraged at their inability to save him (Kübler-Ross' stage of anger[2]). His doctors, in turn, unleash their feelings of inadequacy and frustration upon the psychiatrist, who is then given the difficult task of helping both patient and doctor to face a painful reality. Meeting and living with this challenge is no mean accomplishment.

REFERENCES

1. Eissler KR: The Psychiatrist and the Dying Patient. New York, International Universities Press, 1955

2. Kübler-Ross E: On Death and Dying. New York, Macmillan, 1970
3. Weisman AD, Hackett TP: Predilection to death. Psychosom Med 23: 232, 1961
4. Feifel H (ed): The Meaning of Death. New York, McGraw-Hill, 1959
5. Holland JF: Psychological aspects of cancer. In Holland JF, Frei E III (eds): Cancer Medicine. Philadelphia, Lea & Febiger, 1973, pp. 991–1021
6. LeShan L, LeShan E: Psychotherapy and the patient with a limited life span. Psychiatry 24:318, 1961
7. Norton J: Treatment of a dying patient. Psychoanal Study Child 18:541, 1963
8. Friedman HJ: Physician management of dying patients: an exploration. Psychiatry Med 1:295, 1970
9. Schoenberg B, Carr A: Educating the Health Professional in the Psychosocial Care of the Terminally Ill. Conference of Foundation of Thanatology, New York, 1972
10. Meyer BC: Truth and the physician. Bull NY Acad Med 45:59, 1969
11. Rich I, Kalmanson GM: Attitudes of medical residents toward the dying patient in a general hospital. Postgrad Med 40:A-127, 1966
12. Hicks W, Daniels RS: The dying patient, his physician and the psychiatric consultant. Psychosomatics 9:47, 1968
13. Renneker RE: Countertransference reactions to cancer. Psychosom Med 19:409, 1957
14. Lipowski ZJ: Review of consultation psychiatry and psychosomatic medicine I: general principles. Psychosom Med 29:153, 1967

Part III

The Evolution of a Liaison Program: A Teaching and Clinical Model

Commentary

The overriding goal of the liaison psychiatrist is to foster psychological-mindedness. To do so, he must first accumulate a body of knowledge of the normal psychological reactions to medical illness that can be synthesized and integrated with physiological concepts of disease. Second, he must develop effective methods for the transmission of this holistic amalgam that will reflect his understanding of the anatomy of the teaching hospital. Finally, in order to secure the future of liaison psychiatry, he must conduct research that will yield hard data which will give credibility and substance to his recommendations to other psychiatrists, the medical staff, and the hospital administration.

These efforts must be predicated on his knowledge of the impediments to holistic care in the contemporary teaching hospital. This book began with a description of those variables. Essentially, they can be "boiled down" to deficits in training and systems of patient care. We use coronary heart disease to illustrate the defects in training and their consequences. We turn our attention then to the second impediment—flaws in systems of patient care that stem primarily from the structural aspects of the teaching hospital. The concluding chapter of this book presents a schema for the possible minimization of both these flaws.

Our schema is based on the proposition that the liaison psychiatrist must effect alliances with those members of the medical (or surgical) team who are best able to provide psychological care for the patient. In practice, specialty and individual considerations tend to make certain physicians physically and emotionally unavailable for that task. The fact remains, however, that the physician, regardless of his specialty, is uniquely qualified to allay the patient's fears and anxieties—to help him to cope with the stresses of illness and hospitalization. In the eyes of the patient, the physician is endowed with all-powerful, all-caring capacities; in short, the patient perceives the physician in much the same way as he perceived his parents when he was a child. Whether he wants to or not, the physician cannot ignore this given. Nor can he, in good conscience, delegate responsibility for the psychological well-being of the patient to a staff member who cannot fill that role as effectively. Consequently, the move to the nurse advocated by so many workers in liaison psychiatry does not represent the ideal; nor, in fact, may it even be feasible. The nurse, like the doctor, may not be receptive to psychological data, and her contact may be just as evanescent. On the other hand, a move to the team approach, while born of necessity, may prove useful if the team thereby enables an individual to provide psychological care for the patient. Our quarrel lies with those physicians who cannot even participate in a team effort. Realistic considerations may prevent the doctor from functioning as the primary psychological caretaker, but they do not absolve him from functioning at the next hierarchical level, that is, as chief or leader of the team to provide total care for his patient.

The problem, then, is to induce the doctor to assume some measure of responsibility for the patient's mind and body. We have learned from experience that the usual educational tools, for example, ward rounds, didactic seminars, and curbstone conferences—and even the unusual tools, for example, the Balint seminars described in Chapter 1—are not sufficiently potent to accomplish the task of heightening psychological-mindedness in all physicians, throughout the hospital. The most effective solution seems to us to lie in the liaison psychiatrist's ability to effect an alliance with the hospital administration that will ensure psychological accountability in the ways outlined in the final pages of this book.

Chapter 12

The Liaison Model of Coronary Heart Disease

It is our firm conviction that the liaison psychiatrist's efforts to convince his medical colleagues of the value of psychological intervention must be supported by substantive research and compelling clinical data. Coronary heart disease can be used to demonstrate the need for collaborative observation, intervention, and research on the somatopsychic and psychosomatic phenomena that occur at each of the three phases of an illness: the pre-illness phase, the acute illness phase, and the convalescent phase. Thus, in a larger sense, this chapter can serve as a bridge between the theoretical and clinical material presented in Parts I and II of this book, and the dissemination of this material as elucidated in the following chapters of this section.

In an attempt to clarify the effects of emotions on the cardiovascular system, we begin with a review and evaluation of some of the available psychobiological and clinical research data. We proceed then to a discussion of the clinical implications of these data, and of our own "front line" clinical experience, for the psychological understanding and management of the coronary patient.

PSYCHOBIOLOGICAL AND CLINICAL RESEARCH DATA

Coronary heart disease offers an excellent opportunity to study the effect of psychological stress that stems from physical dysfunction on the one hand and the physical consequences of these psychological reactions on the other.

Predisposing Factors

It is generally felt that certain psychological and physiological phenomena predispose an individual to the development of coronary heart disease. Over the last several years, important, careful, and, at times, ingenious research has been conducted in an attempt to isolate these factors in order to identify persons at risk for this disease. Certain risk factors, such as obesity, smoking, blood triglyceride levels, congenital malformations, diseases like diabetes and hypertension, lack of exercise, and a family history of coronary heart disease seem to be quite soundly implicated. However, our knowledge of psychological risk factors, such as personality type, occupation, stress, and so forth, is less certain, and research in this area has led to the publication of contradictory and confusing data.* For example, the validity of the hypothesis advanced by Friedman and Rosenman[1] that individuals who are well educated, highly competitive, and time-conscious (the "Type A" personality) are predisposed to cardiac disease has been questioned by a number of workers, among them Ostfeld, Lebovits, Shekelle, and Paul.[2] And the findings published by Hinkle, Whitney, Lehmanetal,[3] were diametrically opposed to those of Friedman and Rosenman. Thus Hinkle and his co-workers concluded from their study that highly educated, competitive individuals are less susceptible to coronary disease. However, Jenkins[4] has criticized Hinkle's study on the grounds that the category "highly educated" was not defined with sufficient specificity; nor was any attempt made to differentiate between different types of coronary disease in the patients studied. Jenkins correctly points out that these variables must be taken into account in any study that attempts to identify the psychological and social precursors of coronary disease. Furthermore, social, economic, and ethnic differences in the populations of any study must be considered. For example, Jews have a higher incidence of diabetes (a predisposing factor) and blacks are more likely to have hypertension (a predisposing factor).

* Personality has "reentered" psychosomatic research. Initially the work of Dunbar described global personality types and their relationship to disease. Alexander reported personality characteristics he thought to be associated with specific psychosomatic illnesses and this historical review was sketched in Chapters 1 and 6. In fact in many ways the "Type A" personality described by Friedman and Rosenman[1] is quite similar to that previously ascribed to patients with hypertension or peptic ulcer disease, namely pseudoindependent, striving, driving, competitive, excessively demanding of self and others, etc. Furthermore, it is clear that many patients with coronary heart disease are not "Type A." The important point to learn from history in order to avoid repetitive, nonproductive blind alleys is that personality must be studied along with other physiological and psychological factors, which may then, collectively and/or in relationship to each other, constitute predisposing factors in *some* individuals: A specific personality per se predisposing to a specific physiological disease seems unlikely. (Dr. Herbert Weiner has assisted in this discussion).

Whatever its limitations, the Friedman and Rosenman study constitutes a valuable initial effort to explore the psychobiology of coronary heart disease. Thus the criticisms noted above should be utilized, in our opinion, for the further refinement of similar investigatory efforts. Even if the "Type A" personality is not pathogenic per se, it may be one marker, among others, of a constitutional predisposition to coronary heart disease and, as such, would constitute an important clue that warrants further study.

Some investigators[5] contend that psychological testing can differentiate prospective coronary patients from the general population. Others[2, 6] feel there is no cluster of personality traits that can differentiate prospective coronary patients from the general population. However, Ostfeld and his co-workers[2] reported that individuals who subsequently develop angina score significantly higher on the Hypochondriasis and Hysteria scale when compared with those who develop a coronary thrombosis; the prospective anginal patients also score higher on the Hysteria scale as compared to normals. Furthermore, survivors differed from nonsurvivors on the pre-illness MMPI scale, neurotic triad.[7]

Studies that employ psychological testing present another kind of methodological difficulty. First, testing devices may not probe categories and factors that we feel should be explored, and clearly it is difficult to be quantitative and qualitative at the same time in a sufficiently refined manner. Furthermore, instruments like the MMPI that attempt to "measure" hysteria, a diagnosis, and depression, an affect, describe categories that are essentially not comparable.

It is abundantly clear from this brief review that existing psychological–psychosocial–physiological studies of the etiology of coronary heart disease need to be extended and refined. Weiner's elucidation[8] of the methodological problems that have impeded progress in psychosomatic research has relevance in this context. First, although, as mentioned above, there is substantial agreement as to the physiological factors that predispose an individual to coronary heart disease, our knowledge of these variables is by no means complete. Second, the interrelationship of these physiological risk factors and their relative importance is not clear. Third, although it seems fairly certain that specific psychological factors play a role in the onset of coronary heart disease, they have not been studied in sufficient depth to enable their precise identification. Fourth, the nature of the interrelationship between physiological and psychological factors in coronary heart disease is not understood. And, fifth, we have yet to determine which combinations of these variables are most pernicious in terms of the predisposition to this illness and its initiation.

Reiser[9] has, for some time, urged the refinement of research on coronary heart disease along these lines. Specifically, he has suggested that the physiological factors thought to predispose to this illness, i.e., smoking, hypertension, triglycerides, exercise, and constitution, be studied longitudinally and then compared with psychological risk factors, such as the "Type A" personality described by Rosenman and Friedman,[1] to ascertain their relationship to the occurrence of coronary heart disease.

Other workers have followed other paths of investigation. Rahe, Fløistad, Bergan, and colleagues[10] found that life stresses and life changes heighten the potential for heart attacks and, in fact, for all illness. And Parkes, Benjamin, and Fitzgerald[11] reported that the majority of deaths in the first six months of widowerhood could be accounted for by coronary heart disease. But such research on the role of external psychological events in the onset of coronary heart disease is similarly marred by the methodological defects described above.

Studies of life stresses and the occurrence of coronary heart disease are to date by and large post dictive. Does the life event occur because of the heart disease, e.g. change from a second floor residence because of dyspnea secondary to incipient and as yet unidentified coronary heart disease, or does the heart disease occur because of the life event? Moreover, we do not understand how life stresses and their concomitant affects are translated into physiological dysfunction. Is there a relationship among stress, catecholamines, and the development of arrhythmias, angina, and atheromatous plaques?

Animal studies may provide a breakthrough in this methodological stalemate. Henry, Stephens, Axelrod et al[12] have devised ingenious experiments in mice that clearly show the relationship between psychosocial stress, namely crowding, and physiological changes, including subsequent increased adrenal weight, increased tyrosine hydroxylase (the rate-limiting enzyme in norepinephrine synthesis), renal pathology, and sustained hypertension, which can lead to death. However, recent studies have underscored the danger of prematurely ascribing physiological changes to psychosocial events. For example, Hofer and Weiner[13] found that early separation of the rat pup from its mother produced a predisposition to irregular heart rate and rhythm and increased lability of blood pressure. Initially, these physiological phenomena were interpreted as a consequence of separation from the mother per se. However, it subsequently became apparent that it was the lack of milk supplied by the mother rather than the unavailability of the object (mother) that was the critical variable for the decrease in heart rate.

Initiating Factors and Mechanisms

There is compelling evidence that emotions, and anxiety in particular, increase cardiac work. For example, Hickam, Cargill, and Golden[14] concluded from their study of the cardiac function of normal students undergoing the stress of college examinations that anxiety, like exertion, increases cardiac output. It follows, then, that in a delicately compensated, diseased heart, anxiety can lead to coronary insufficiency and heart failure. The description by Chambers and Reiser[15] of emotional events that had occurred in their subjects prior to the onset of congestive heart failure suggests that affects played a role in the exacerbation of the disease. And EKG changes and a decrease in functional cardiac reserve were shown to occur with tension.

It has been suggested that cardiac function can also be affected by moods. According to Stein,[16] gloomy patients in a coronary care unit had increased morbidity. And Cassem and Hackett[17] found that the mortality rate from coronary disease was significantly diminished in patients in a coronary care unit referred for psychiatric consultation. Actually, the meaning of the findings derived from both these studies is uncertain. (1) It may be that patients with mood disturbance (e.g., gloom) are sicker and their more severe illness results in poorer outcome, with psychological concomitants a correlated phenomenon. However, such a finding would still identify a high-risk group that should be studied to learn if psychological intervention does affect outcome. (2) Certain methodological problems must be resolved if decreased mortality is used as an index of the effectiveness of psychiatric intervention. For example, in our coronary care unit at Montefiore the overall death rate is only about 9 percent without routine psychiatric consultation. To show a significant reduction in mortality, one would require a large sample gathered over time. One would have to control for the therapeutic effects of increased experience acquired by the medical staff during this period, for technological advances in patient care that might be introduced, and for changes in the severity of the illness of the population studied. Since Cassem and Hackett did not control for these variables, their findings are not conclusive.

The relationship between physiological and psychological factors persists during the convalescent phase of coronary heart disease, and now manifests itself in mood disorders and phobias and inhibitions surrounding sex and work.

It is generally agreed that most coronary patients are medically able to return to sex approximately six weeks after their attack. However, a large percentage of this group have a delayed return to sex, or engage in sexual intercourse with greatly decreased frequency, or become impotent.

Croog, Levine, and Lurie[18] deplore the absence of research that would facilitate identification of the patient who will have sexual problems once he leaves the hospital. One exemplary study has been conducted in this area, however, by Hellerstein and Friedman.[19]

These authors conducted an investigation of the sexual functioning of a group of 91 males, consisting of 48 postcoronary patients and 43 normal persons, which incorporated the use of EKG monitoring at the subject's place of work and at home in the privacy of his bedroom. Hellerstein and Friedman posed the following important questions: (1) What is the actual magnitude of the strain on the heart during marital intercourse? (2) Can the anxiety that is partially responsible for increased cardiac work during sexual intercourse be modified through counseling? (3) What are the psychological determinants of the coronary patient's future sexual adjustment?

The study findings yielded the answer to the first question: the magnitude of the strain on the heart of sexual intercourse in long-married couples (as measured by oxygen cost) was equivalent to the strain of climbing a flight of stairs, walking briskly, or performing the routine tasks involved in many occupations, and less than that required to perform a standard single master two-step test.* Apparently, however, extramarital coitus was more stressful: 80 percent of the reported coital deaths occurred under these circumstances.

In the group studied by Hellerstein and Friedman, on the average, sexual activity was not resumed until fourteen weeks postcoronary. And, not surprisingly, the physiologically symptomatic patients were the most reluctant to resume sexual intercourse. Furthermore, two-thirds of the patients studied engaged in sex less frequently after their coronary attack. Interestingly, most of these patients ascribed this change to their decreased sexual desire or their wives' fears. They did not mention coronary symptoms as a causative factor; nor did they claim that their physicians had prohibited sexual activity. But, in fact, increased blood pressure and cardiac symptoms were correlated with a decrease in the frequency of postcoronary sexual activity in this patient group six months after an attack. On the other hand, at one year postcoronary, by which time the sexual phobia had consolidated, physical factors did not correlate with a decrease in frequency of coital episodes.

Unfortunately, Hellerstein and Friedman do not describe their intractable patients who remained fearful of ever resuming sexual intercourse. Moreover, none of the postcoronary subjects studied by Hellerstein and Friedman said they were impotent, which is in sharp contrast to the findings reported by Weiss and English[20] who described impotence as the most frequent sexual problem in postcoronary patients. And Tuttle, Cook, and Fitch[21] reported that 10 percent of their research sample had developed permanent psychogenic impotence after their coronary attack.

---

* Hellerstein and Friedman suggest that the prophylactic precoital use of nitroglycerine can improve sexual performance in patients who experience angina, and thereby improve attitudes toward sexual intercourse.

In contrast to the paucity of psychobiological and clinical research on the sexual functioning of the postcoronary patient, the work inhibitions of this patient group have been studied extensively. Croog and his co-workers[18] concluded from their review of the literature that approximately 20 percent of all postcoronary patients do not return to work, despite the fact that they are physiologically able to do so and have received medical assurance to that effect. They also point out that there is some evidence that rehabilitation programs have enabled more patients to return to work, but the studies of such programs involved small groups of patients and were not well controlled.

Zohman's study[22] at Montefiore cannot be criticized on these methodological grounds. She attempted to determine why some patients are able to go back to work two to three months after a coronary, while others take a year to do so, and still others never go back. The recalcitrant patient's attitude toward work was related to several issues: persistent cardiac symptoms and inadequate physical conditioning for job functioning; psychological issues, as these emerged in test findings (e.g., a questionnaire assessment and the rod and frame objective test); vocational reasons (a need for job modification); and socioeconomic factors (the availability of welfare payments and disability insurance, so that work was not a financial imperative).

Zohman attempted to counteract these patients' failure to return to work by offering them social and recreational outlets, exercise, and simulated on-the-job training, with EKG radiotelemetry. In addition, psychological counseling was done in groups, led by a social worker; in this setting the patients and their wives were able to express their mutual anxieties.

The patients who participated in this program were then compared to a control group of postcoronary patients who had psychological evaluation only. The results on vocational outcome showed that the patients in the experimental group returned to work—and to the same job—more frequently at three to six months than did the control group, but the difference was not statistically significant. And at one year the groups were not distinguishable.

CLINICAL IMPLICATIONS

The methodological and conceptual problems inherent in these psychobiological and clinical research efforts restrict the amount of meaningful clinical data available to internists and cardiologists. Therefore, this discussion of the signs and symptoms of psychological dysfunction in the coronary patient and their management is based primarily on our "front line" experience; the research findings presented earlier provide guidelines and useful adjuncts for diagnosis and intervention in coronary heart disease during the acute and convalescent phases of the illness.

Coronary heart disease can serve as a model of the psychological reactions evoked by an acute medical illness in the "normal" patient. All seven of the basic psychological stresses enumerated in Chapter 3, including the threat to narcissistic integrity, fear of strangers, separation anxiety, fear of loss of love and approval, fear of loss of control, castration anxiety, and reactivation of feelings of guilt and shame, are apparent as one listens to these patients.

However, some stresses are more prominent than others at different periods in the course of the illness, and management techniques and goals differ accordingly. As noted earlier, the stresses that are prominent during the pre-illness phase have not yet been identified.* Therefore, for purposes of this discussion, coronary heart disease has been conceptualized as consisting of two phases: the acute illness phase and the convalescent phase.

At each phase we have identified the psychological tags (symptoms, character reactions, and so on, that derive from the seven basic psychological stresses) that can serve as clues to the patient's need for psychological intervention. The formulation of these tags and of the prescribed interventions was based on the principles of psychoanalytic psychology, and the theories of ego psychology in particular.

Acute Illness Phase

Catalog of Psychological Tags. The patient's specific responses to his illness relate to his premorbid conflicts, previous hospital experiences, the meaning the illness holds for him, and his relationship to early caretakers (parents). Thus his behavior may stem from fears of dependency, excessive fears of bodily damage, fear of the loss of sexual identity (i.e., that he will be "half a man" after he leaves the hospital), or perception of his illness as punishment. And, finally, out of a sense of guilt, he may identify with someone he was close to who had a coronary and died.

Since the illness has an acute onset, it may overwhelm the patient,

---

* In any event, at present, the liaison psychiatrist does research, but, of course, does not treat patients at risk for coronary heart disease. We would hope, however, that as research into the etiology of this disease uncovers psychological risk factors, the psychiatrist will be given an opportunity to help the internist to identify vulnerable individuals, and to recommend appropriate prophylactic measures. Ideally, the hospital would then organize its facilities to incorporate a treatment unit for the pre-illness phase (primary prevention), similar to the units that are now available for the acute phase, and are provided by some teaching hospitals (e.g., Montefiore Hospital) for the posthospital convalescent phase of the disease.

leaving him confused, panic-stricken, and numbed. He may defend against these feelings in a variety of ways, and develop behavioral reactions—specifically, anxiety reactions, depressive reactions, and exaggerated character traits (e.g., belligerence)—that ultimately put more stress on his heart. Regardless of their nature, if the patient's maladaptive reactions are not dealt with early in his hospital stay, they may lead to a worsening of his cardiac status or to a permanent psychological dysfunction.

Anxiety: Signs and symptoms of significant anxiety may include difficulty in falling asleep, restlessness, sweating, dry mouth, pressured speech, frequency of urination, and increased pulse rate. The patient may also complain of palpitation, a feeling of impending doom, generalized fatigue, vague aches and pains, shortness of breath (especially a sighing respiration), paresthesia, and have a constant need for reassurance. All of these reactions must be differentiated from the physical effects of the coronary attack and from the effects of the medication the patient is receiving, and must be further differentiated from the symptoms of an organic brain syndrome.

Frequently, the patient is afraid to fall asleep. He may fantasize, for example, that his heart "won't work" unless he monitors it, or that the monitor will electrocute him while he's sleeping. He may dread weekends and nights when his regular physician is off duty, and there may be an exacerbation of his psychological symptoms at these times because he believes no one else "knows" his case.

Depression: Tags suggesting depressive disorders include tearfulness; psychomotor retardation (or agitation); sleep difficulty, with early morning awakening; loss of appetite; feelings of helplessness or hopelessness; suicidal thoughts; and excessive fears of dying. Also important are excessive somatic complaints, for example, gastrointestinal complaints, constipation, and so forth.

Character reactions: Patients who do not like to be confined or told what to do represent potential psychological risks. The patient who boasts that he has "never been sick a day in his life," who "doesn't believe in doctors," who takes pride in being his "own boss," and who says he "could never work for anyone," may very well become a management problem. Equally important are data suggesting a marked tendency toward nonverbal discharge of tension. Thus, such a patient might say, "I'm always on the go; I can't sit still," or "I get depressed on Sundays and when I'm on vacation."

The patient's anxiety, depression, and character reactions may all interfere with his psychological comfort, physiological status, and his medical management. For example, such a patient may sign out of the hospital, or refuse prescribed medication. On the other hand, the absence of some anxiety or depression in a patient may be a tag of highly defended fears and anxieties that are just as pernicious.

Interventions. In general, given the interrelationship that exists between psychological and biological factors, particularly during the acute illness phase of coronary heart disease, it seems evident that an anxious patient in the coronary care unit should have psychological, psychopharmacological, and environmental intervention as indicated.

Our primary goal at this phase is symptom reduction (secondary prevention). This can be accomplished by two approaches: psychopharmacological intervention is used to alleviate disturbing affects; psychological intervention is directed toward reducing the patient's symptoms by uncovering their source and, at the same time, strengthening the patient's ability to cope with his distress. In addition, we alert the medical team in the coronary care unit to the patient's psychological distress, its probable source, and the significance of the psychological symptom for his immediate well-being, as well as his recovery and convalescence. And we attempt to instruct the patient's medical caretakers in the use of psychological and psychopharmacological therapeutic techniques.

> Mr. L., a 53-year-old engineer, had sustained a myocardial infarction one year prior to his current hospitalization for arrhythmia. A psychiatric consultation was requested after he became panic-stricken following the insertion of a temporary pacemaker. Mr. L. felt "like a robot whose heart had been replaced by a machine," and experienced diffuse chest pain. But there were no EKG changes. The doctors felt that Mr. L. was overconcerned about his pacemaker, and questioned the reality of his physical distress.
>
> The psychiatrist found that Mr. L. was quite anxious. He sat up frequently, and sweated profusely. He expressed anger at the staff because he felt they minimized his physical problems and therefore were not giving him the care he needed. At the same time, he was afraid that his anger would accelerate the pacemaker and that he would be electrocuted. With some hesitation, he wondered aloud, "If I have sex, will the same thing happen? You know I had this attack after a terrible fight with my wife. Then I took her to bed so we could make up, like we usually do. I know that if I have a sexual feeling now, I'll die. If I look at a pretty girl, I'll die too. But how can you be a man and not look at a pretty girl?"
>
> Mr. L. described his heart attack and subsequent arrythmia as "crippling blows." He had always been an active man—and his own man. Now his whole life had changed. His wife had taken over; she had returned to work, chauffeured him around, and in essence wore the pants. On the day he had his attack of arrhythmia, he had become enraged at her "bossy" attitude.

The insertion of the pacemaker stimulated Mr. L.'s fears of being dependent on anyone or anything, and, on a deeper level, his passive feminine fears. Mr. L. considered help an intrusion. Thus he deeply resented having "to be driven" by a pacemaker—or having to be driven by his wife. On the other hand, the failure of his doctors to respond to his need was an abandonment. He felt depressed, weak, powerless, damaged—and angry. But he was afraid that if he lost control of his anger, his bodily functions and the pacemaker would go out of control too, and he would be electrocuted. His rage was projected in part onto the pacemaker, which would take over and destroy him in retaliation for his anger, which he felt he had to curb at all costs.

Mr. L. had other fears of bodily damage. In his mind, his heart, as a vital organ, was equated with his vital sexual organ, so that the death of his heart's functioning was equated with sexual death, and resulted in paralyzing anxiety.

Psychopharmacological, psychological, and environmental interventions were used in this case.

Psychopharmacological intervention: Valium is routinely used for patients in the coronary care unit. However, other drugs, such as the phenothiazines, which can be used safely in coronary heart disease, may be more potent anti-anxiety agents (see Chapter 9). Thus Stelazine, which was prescribed for Mr. L., provided tranquilization without producing drowsiness, which would have made him more anxious, for in a drowsy state he would have felt more vulnerable and less in control.

Psychological intervention: We offered Mr. L. supportive therapy by encouraging him to ventilate his anger at the doctors who "didn't take him seriously." And we encouraged his doctors to express their annoyance with Mr. L. for complaining so much. Only after Mr. L. had verbalized his rage did he realize that it was not physically destructive, and would not provoke retaliation from others. In addition, the doctors were helped to understand that accepting Mr. L.'s feelings, but setting limits at the same time, would reduce his anxiety. The connection between Mr. L.'s behavior toward the staff and his behavior toward his wife was clarified by the psychiatrist: Mr. L. was told that when he felt dependent on the staff or his wife, it was necessary for him to assert himself by fighting with them or her in order to feel "manly." This led to the insight that he was not being "rejected" by his wife and the staff. Rather, it was he who, because of his own fears, was keeping away the people he really needed and wanted.

Mr. L. feared that physical as well as emotional activity would damage his heart, and he was reassured on both scores by "scientific" means. Specifically, we monitored all his activities (e.g., yelling, being angry, crying, walking, and climbing stairs) by portable EKG, and showed him that they were safe. He was also told that when he returned home, his sexual activity could be monitored in the same way. Furthermore, he began to perceive the pacemaker as an ally, rather than as an internal destructive force. Finally, we dealt directly with Mr. L.'s pathogenic fantasy that his heart attack had damaged his maleness and that his vital organs would not work without an outside power.

Environmental manipulation: We utilized Mr. L.'s engineering background to reinforce his intellectual defenses and mastery. Thus, for example, he was encouraged to explain how the electronic devices in the coronary care unit, including the pacemaker, worked to the other patients. His efforts to identify with his doctors produced feelings of satisfaction and increased his self-esteem. (They also reduced his doctors' annoyance with him.)

Convalescent Phase

Catalog of Psychological Tags. The most prominent psychological tags during the convalescent phase are phobias or inhibitions relating to work or sex; depression; fear of being alone; hypochondriacal fears, which need not necessarily center on the heart; and the somatization of anxiety, which would include palpitation, dyspnea, excessive fatigue, and chest pains, all of which may convince the patient that he is having another heart attack. These symptoms may be a response to the reality of new adaptational stresses that arise during the convalescent phase; or they may be manifestations of the persistent pathogenic fantasies that were precipitated by the coronary attack.

Interventions. Psychological intervention during this phase is governed by the goals of tertiary prevention:

1. To prevent a recurrence of the physiological disease by reducing stress.
2. To prevent the occurrence or exacerbation of psychological dysfunction by dealing with the patient's inhibitions and phobias surrounding work and sex, as well as his postcoronary psychological symptoms, such as depression and the somatization of anxiety.
3. To help the patient to adapt to his physiological and psychological limitations.

We attempt to implement these goals by alerting the physician to the psychological factors that may be impeding the patient's recovery, by educating the physician with respect to their management, and by alerting him to the use of specific highly efficient physiologic tools that can facilitate his efforts to this end. The development of sophisticated technology, for example, EKG radiotelemetry and micromapping of cardiac ischemia, means that the magnitude of strain on the heart caused by work and sexual activities can be assessed precisely and demonstrated, which should be reassuring for many anxious patients. Once the patient is confronted with proof that he is, in fact, physiologically capable of resuming these activities, the anxiety that has inhibited his return to work and/or sex, or, more specifically, the malignant fantasies that have given rise to this anxiety can be dealt with directly.

The three cases described below are representative of the spectrum of postcoronary convalescent problems, ranging from mild psychopathology (greater recovery potential) to often irreversible psychopathology, commonly encountered in this patient population.

> Mr. V., a 43-year-old truck driver, was admitted to the hospital with a coronary attack. Further medical evaluation revealed hypertension and incipient heart failure. The patient responded well medically, and was discharged to the Work Rehabilitation Unit and Coronary Experimental Drug Project at Montefiore. In the Work Rehabilitation Unit, Mr. V. was monitored by EKG telemetry, which showed severe ischemic changes while he loaded boxes on a truck (which was one of the routine tasks he would be expected to perform if he returned to his old job). Consequently, his doctor was against his returning to his work. In the Coronary Experimental Drug Project he was told he would be given one of three drugs, and he learned that estrogen, which could cause mammary development, was included among them.* Although Mr. V. was not told which specific drug he was given, he was convinced he was receiving estrogen compounds.
>
> Mr. V. was seen by a psychiatrist six months after his coronary as part of a hospital study. He admitted that he was anxious and depressed because, he explained, he could not perform sexually. Although he felt aroused, he was afraid to "try" with his wife. He talked about his previous active sexual life, and confessed to an extramarital affair, which he felt was linked to his heart attack. The psychiatrist also learned that he had stopped taking the experimental drug after one week, because he felt it made him "chesty like a woman."
>
> Mr. V. was also depressed because he had been told he could not return to his old job. He was proud of driving the "big rigs," of being the "top banana," and could not see himself behind a desk. He boasted that even if his heart stopped while he was driving, he could thump his own chest. In fact, he had returned to his old job, without telling his doctor. Nor had he told his doctor that he had stopped taking the drug. Furthermore, Mr. V.'s physician was not

---

* This is standard procedure. All patients in the Drug Project are told they will be receiving one of three drugs, the names of the drugs, and the possible side effects of each, in conformance with standards of patient consent that must be adhered to in all studies of human subjects.

aware of the fact that his patient felt his extramarital affair was the
direct precipitant of his heart attack, and that this was the reason
he was afraid to "try sex" again.

Mr. V. had two symptoms—a phobic avoidance of sex and a tendency to
defend against anxiety by overcompensation. It was an interesting paradox
that he felt that hard physical work would not damage his heart but that sex
would. This paradox can be explained, in part, by the fact that Mr. V.
consciously viewed his illness as a punishment for his extramarital affair,
and used his abstinence to punish himself further. His unrealistic desire to
return to work was still a third, albeit less conscious, expression of his
need for punishment. Thus Mr. V. was vaguely aware of the self-destructive motives that governed his behavior, but he was powerless to change.

However, he was completely unaware of the defensive aspects of his
behavior. On the basis of our interviews with Mr. V., we concluded that
he equated his heart attack with (imagined) damage to his masculinity,*
which had been reinforced by the real physiological changes induced by
the estrogen. (Mr. V. had received an estrogen drug.) Thus his determination to avoid a passive posture, which would include sitting behind a desk
or submitting to a doctor's orders, was a defense against the anxiety provoked by this fantasied emasculation. His compulsive need to drive the
"big rigs" and be the "top banana" were additional restitutive maneuvers.

The psychiatrist attempted to deal with Mr. V.'s maladaptive, but ultimately tractable, posthospital convalescent problems in several ways. His
overall goals were to reduce Mr. V.'s psychological symptoms and help
him to adapt realistically to his disability, and in this instance he was able
to involve the cardiologist in the pursuit of these goals.

Obviously, it would not have been feasible in this setting to explore the
roots of Mr. V.'s passive feminine concerns. Instead, we relied on supportive therapy, and attempted to bolster his sense of masculinity. For example, the cardiologist was advised and agreed to give Mr. V. a realistic
voice in the management of his illness. The estrogens were not reintro-
duced. In fact, the cardiologist was urged to eschew any drug or intervention that would make the patient feel weak or helpless. After Mr. V.'s
anxiety was reduced, he consented to undergo vocational training for
another job in the trucking field—and subsequently accepted a position as
a dispatcher, where he was able to give orders to the other truckers.

Mr. V. was reassured that there was no relationship between his
extramarital affair and his heart attack, which reduced his feelings of
guilt. As a result, he no longer had to punish himself by abstaining from

---

* The scope of these interviews was necessarily limited. Thus, for example, we did
not elicit a detailed account from Mr. V. of his childhood history, which, of course,
would have enabled confirmation of our formulations.

sex. In addition, the cardiologist's reassurance that sex per se could not cause a heart attack reduced his general concern about sex. Finally, he was "monitored' by remote EKG to further reassure him that sex would not be harmful to his heart.

EKG monitoring was also used to convince Mr. V. that his old job was dangerous. When he experienced chest pains while driving his truck, and could actually see these changes on a portable EKG, this reinforced his decision to accept a less physically demanding job.

In contrast to Mr. V., Mr. W. had a work phobia, and was unable to resolve this problem.

> Mr. W., who had sustained a myocardial infarction at the age of 48, was, like Mr. V., a truck driver. His hospital stay was marked by vituperative and self-destructive behavior; for example, he smoked three to four packs of cigarettes a day and refused to stay in bed. Like Mr. V., Mr. W. was assigned to the Work Rehabilitation Unit after he was discharged from the hospital, and was given on-the-job monitoring. But unlike Mr. V., he showed no EKG changes with heavy work, and was reassured that he could return to his regular job as a driver.
>
> When Mr. W. was seen by his cardiologist several months after he had been discharged from the hospital, he reported that he had resumed his normal sexual life. But he admitted that he had not returned to work and explained, matter-of-factly, that he had only "25 percent horsepower left," and didn't "want to take unnecessary risks." When his cardiologist confronted him with the reality of his physical condition, that is, the mildness of his heart attack and his full recovery, he retorted that doctors were not infallible.
>
> Apparently, Mr. W.'s daily routine consisted of feeding his rabbits, sitting in the sun, and gossiping with his friends. He explained his "philosophy" to his cardiologist. Quite simply, he felt he had been "struck down" in his prime because he had worked so hard all his life. Now he was "entitled" to sit back and collect disability insurance.

In direct contrast to Mr. V., Mr. W. was concerned about the physical consequences of hard work, rather than of sexual activity. However, the illness held similar unconscious psychological meanings for both patients. That is, as was true of Mr. V., Mr. W.'s heart attack stimulated intense castration anxiety (i.e., now he only had "25 percent horsepower left"). Thus, although Mr. W. appeared to function well sexually, actually, his vigorous sexual activity was, in part, a defense against his intense fear and denial of bodily damage. On the other hand, his fear of bodily damage prevented him from returning to work. His belligerent behavior during the acute phase of his illness can be understood, in retrospect, as an early indication of his need to defend against his imagined loss of masculinity.

Consciously, Mr. W. felt that hard work and his aggressive, ambitious attitude had caused his heart attack. Thus, apart from the fact that his work phobia stemmed from his need to defend against his fear of bodily damage, it can be speculated that this specific symptom served to resolve many conflicts centering around aggression, competitiveness, and the fear of retaliation.

Finally, Mr. W.'s non-return to work can also be explained, in part, by his strong, previously unfulfilled and warded-off dependency needs that could now be legitimately gratified. Thus Mr. W.'s work phobia was further reinforced by his disability insurance payments and his wife's protective attitude toward him (secondary gain).

Mr. W. was seen once by the psychiatrist, but he refused to continue treatment, and his cardiologist did not press him to do so. The cardiologist agreed with Björck[23] that this type of patient should not be forced to go back to work. And, in this instance, the psychiatrist was unable to convince either the cardiologist or the patient that the failure to return to work was, at base, a major psychological symptom that might respond to treatment.

The third patient, described below, is typical of the true cardiac cripple.

> Mr. Q. had a history of rheumatic heart disease with valvular damage since childhood. When he was 44 years old he was operated on and a valvular prosthesis was inserted.
>
> Prior to his operation, Mr. Q. had received social security disability payments. He had never worked; nor had he ever married. He lived with his elderly parents. Although catheter and clinical studies showed marked cardiovascular improvement postoperatively, Mr. Q. continued to complain of incapacitating dyspnea and fatigue. In short, he continued to be an invalid.

Mr. Q.'s life-long cardiac status had become an integral part of him, and this psychological component was not removed by surgery. Consequently, he did not show psychological improvement postoperatively, commensurate with his physiological improvement.

The cardiologist and psychiatrist agreed that because Mr. Q.'s character structure and self-image as a helpless cardiac cripple were fixed, his work and sex potential were extremely limited. In fact, he developed additional psychological symptoms—anxiety, guilt, and depression—postoperatively because the dramatic change in his life style that he and others expected did not materialize. These postoperative symptoms lessened somewhat when Mr. Q. was "reassured" (and his family was advised) that he was not expected to change his life style, and that his disability insurance would be continued. His anxiety, depression, and guilt about his inability to function were then relieved. But these symptoms might not have appeared in the first place if the cardiologist and the psychiatrist had prepared Mr. Q. preoperatively for the possibility that his physiological improvement would not immediately carry with it corresponding improvements in his work and sexual functioning.

The three patients discussed here were cared for primarily by their cardiologists; in our opinion, only one, Mr. V., received adequate psychological care. We were not given an opportunity to try to help Mr. W., and we were not asked to see Mr. Q. preoperatively, when he could have benefited most from psychological intervention.

SUMMARY AND CONCLUSIONS

Our "front line" clinical experience with coronary patients, and the findings yielded to date by psychobiological and clinical research on coronary heart disease, clearly attest to the need for psychological diagnosis and intervention during the acute and convalescent phases of the illness. Unfortunately, however, cardiologists and internists are drawn to one superficial aspect of psychobiological research—anxiety increases cardiac work—and their interventions may therefore be limited to the control of affects by the blanket use of reassurance and/or medication. They are not able to individualize or sufficiently pursue the sources of the patient's psychological distress.

Why is it so important for the physician to recognize the importance of psychological factors at each phase of the illness, to identify their source, and to apply appropriate interventions?

All medical illnesses evoke the seven basic psychological stresses, and this is no less true of coronary heart disease. However, we have been impressed by the frequency with which derivatives of these stresses occur in these patients, and by the prominence, in particular, of derivatives of castration anxiety. There is an unconscious symbolic equation that a damaged body, that is, a damaged heart = a damaged self, that is, damaged genitals = death.* We know, too, that even when there is no overt manifestation of this anxiety, it may be present nonetheless throughout the acute

---

* This observation is limited, in the main, to our experience with male coronary patients. It may be that it would apply to women as well, although we would expect the derivatives to be different. Unfortunately, investigators of both the psychobiological and psychological aspects of coronary heart disease have not addressed themselves to the psychological problems of female coronary patients, and we are guilty of the same omission.

phase of the disease, and that if it is not dealt with, it can persist during the convalescent phase and lead to the development of fixed psychological dysfunction—work and/or sex inhibitions or chronic psychological symptoms. Certainly the prospect of this outcome should convince the physician of the need to recognize and deal with his patients' psychological problems.

At any given phase of the illness, there may be discordance between the patient's reactions to his heart disease and the physician's understanding of these reactions. Thus, first and foremost, the psychiatrist must foster the physician's deeper understanding of the patient's communications during the acute phase of his illness. No physician is unfamiliar with the litany of the male coronary patient: "Doctor will I work again?" "Is my body going to be alright?" "Will I be a whole man?" "Can I live a normal life?" "Will I be my old self?" These questions convey deeper worries that often go unheeded. But these worries cannot be dealt with effectively unless the physician is willing to actively pursue the source of the patient's anxiety, to ask questions that will elicit fantasy material. The physician must recognize the significance of these fantasies if he is to deal with them.

As the patient recovers physically, the physician is confronted with an individual whose physical complaints become increasingly diffuse and, in fact, represent his persistent worries about the intactness of his self and his capacity to perform. Yet, once again, patient and physician communicate on a superficial level, and on a level that is inappropriate to the phase of the illness. Even when the patient's psychological distress is evident, that is, when he reports a work or sex inhibition, the physician is reluctant to deal with the patient's problem himself or in conjunction with a psychiatrist.

In fact, cardiologists and internists have shown a marked resistance to date to the acceptance and application of psychological formulations. Consequently, if the psychiatrist is to expand the physician's armamentarium, he must also identify the cause of this resistance and try to overcome it. It can be speculated, for example, that the physician's unconscious image of himself as a destructive force, as described by Spikes and Holland in Chapter 11, may be responsible, in part, for his belief that if he asks the patient "intimate" questions about sex and death, he will arouse anxiety that will endanger the patient's physical status.

Our task as liaison psychiatrists is threefold: to foster self-awareness in the physician, so that he can work through the internal obstacles (whatever their unconscious source) that may impede his psychological care of the patient; to help him to understand the interplay and relative importance of psychological and physiological factors in coronary heart disease, and, in fact, in any medical illness; and, finally, to provide him with the tools that will enable him to deal effectively with his patient's psychological problems. This is the *raison d'être* for this book.

REFERENCES

1. Friedman M, Rosenman RH: Association of specific overt behavior patterns with blood and cardiovascular findings. JAMA 169:1286–1296, 1950
2. Ostfeld AM, Lebovits BZ, Shekelle RB, Paul O: A prospective study of the relationship between personality and coronary heart disease. J Chronic Dis 17:265–276, 1964
3. Hinkle LE, Whitney LH, Lehman EW, et al: Occupation, education and coronary heart disease. Science 161:238–246, 1968
4. Jenkins CD: Psychologic and social precursors of coronary disease. N Eng J Med 284:244–255, 1971
5. Friedman GD, Ury HK, Klatsky AL, et al: A psychological questionnaire predictive of M.I. Psychosom Med 36:327–343, 1974
6. Mordkoff AM, Parsons OA: The coronary personality: a critique. Psychosom Med 29:1–14, 1967
7. Shekelle RB, Ostfeld AM: Psychometric evaluations in cardiovascular epidemiology. Ann NY Acad Sci 126:696–705, 1965
8. Weiner H: Current status and future prospects for research in psychosomatic medicine. J Psychiat Res 8:479–498, 1971
9. Reiser MF: Changing theoretical concepts in psychosomatic medicine. In Arieti S (ed): The American Handbook of Psychiatry, Vol. IV. New York: Basic Books (in press)
10. Rahe RH, Fløistad I, Bergan T, et al: A model for life changes and illness research. Arch Gen Psychiatry 31:172–177, 1974
11. Parkes CM, Benjamin B, Fitzgerald RG: "Broken heart": a statistical study of increased mortality among widowers. Bri Med J 1:740–743, 1969
12. Henry JP, Stephens PM, Axelrod J, et al: Effect of psychosocial stimulation on the enzymes involved in the biosynthesis and metabolism of noradrenaline and adrenaline. Psychosom Med 33:227–237, 1971
13. Hofer MA, Weiner H: Development of mechanisms of cardiorespiratory responses to maternal deprivation in rat pups. Psychosom Med 33:353–362, 1971
14. Hickam JB, Cargill WH, Golden A: Cardiovascular reactions to emotional stimuli: effect on cardial output, A-V O_2 difference, arterial pressure, and peripheral resistance. J Clin Invest 27:290–298, 1948
15. Chambers W, Reiser MF: Emotional stress in the precipitation of congestive heart failure. Psychosom Med 15:38–60, 1953
16. Stein MJ: Psychosocial Response of Patients: Post-Myocardial Infarction. American Psychosomatic Meetings, Philadelphia, 1974
17. Cassem NH, Hackett TP: Psychiatric consultation in a coronary care unit. Ann Intern Med 75:9–14, 1971
18. Croog SH, Levine S, Lurie Z: The heart patient and the recovery process. Soc Sci Med 2:111–164, 1968
19. Hellerstein HK, Friedman EH: Sexual activity and the post-coronary patient. Arch Intern Med 125:987–999, 1970
20. Weiss E, English OS: Psychosomatic Medicine, 3rd ed. Philadelphia: Saunders, 1957
21. Tuttle WB, Cook WL, Fitch E: Sexual behavior in post-myocardial infarction patients. Am J Cardiol 13:140, 1964

22. Zohman L: Rehabilitating the coronary patient for work. Final Report, Grant RD 1994 M, 1970
23. Björck G: The return to work of patients with myocardial infarction. J Chronic Dis 17:653–657, 1964

Chapter 13

The Anatomy of the Teaching Hospital

James J. Strain

The lack of psychological patient care can, at base, be attributed to two interrelated variables. The first is the lack of viable relationships between and among individuals, that is, the doctor and his patients. The second is the failure of the hospital administration to provide a viable structure and organization that permit adequate psychological care for its patient population. Implicit in Chapter 12 is the notion that the knowledge and skills of the liaison psychiatrist will lie fallow unless he is able to build effective alliances with the medical staff of various hospital departments and services. The thesis of this chapter is that the efforts of the liaison psychiatrist to foster holistic patient care are equally contingent on the psychiatrist's ability to identify and eliminate those defects in the structure and organization of the hospital, which, by their very nature, preclude psychological care of the patient.

The description here of the anatomy of a particular teaching hospital, Montefiore Hospital and Medical Center, necessarily underscores the defects in the structure and organization at that institution. But Montefiore is not unique in this respect. Such deficits are typical of the organization and structure of many, if not most, teaching hospitals.*

The basic flaw in the structure of the contemporary teaching hospital is that its policies and practices are dictated by three disparate and discordant elements: an advisory bureaucracy, multiple conflicting goals, and a need for mechanized patterns of patient care. Each one of these elements is enough, in itself, to detract from the psychological climate essential to

---

* What is more important and must be emphasized in this context is the fact that our report is based on data obtained when our study was initiated in 1968. Since that time, partly as a result of our study, the hospital's administrators, as well as its various departments, have attempted to correct these deficits and have implemented many of the recommendations set forth in Chapter 14.

holistic patient care. Their combined effect is devastating for the quality of clinical services.

The teaching hospital is organized along the lines of an advisory bureaucracy, in which each department is conceived of as a fiefdom (the "comb" effect). Clearly, an advisory bureaucracy is not conducive to the formation of a cohesive unit, and neither the hospital in general, nor the ward in particular can be so characterized. Policies and procedures that govern the operation of the hospital are formulated by lay directors under the guidance of the professionals who head these fiefdoms, and whose primary concern is the autonomy and aggrandizement of their "territory."

Within this operational framework, the administrative policies and practices of the teaching hospital are designed to implement the three prescribed, albeit conflicting, goals of such institutions: to offer optimal clinical services, to provide clinical training in a variety of specialties and subspecialties, and to foster medical research. But the hospital's overriding goal is to fulfill the community's medical needs. Shorter hospital stays, secondary to improved inpatient and outpatient care, earlier diagnosis, and a greater staff and patient tolerance for recuperation at home have made it possible for Montefiore to double its admission rate in the last five years. For example, 100 to 120 patients are presently admitted to a 40-bed unit on the medical ward each month, or an average of 4 to 5 new patients a day. Consequently, despite an augmentation of house staff and special nursing teams, the amount of time a caretaker can spend with any single patient is necessarily limited.

Shorter hospital stays also mean that patients undergo a greater number of diagnostic procedures and examinations per day. As a result, they spend more time away from the ward—away from the physicians and nurses with whom they have established contact, however limited, and from their fellow patients.

In any event, the technological advances that have shortened the duration of hospitalization have created a mechanized environment that is antithetical to the formation of a viable doctor–patient relationship—the crux of good medical practice.

LIFE ON THE WARD

The procedure that has had the most pervasive influence on the climate of the ward and its operation is the system of rotations. The rotation of house doctors, attendings, and nurses is justified on the grounds that it ensures exposure to a variety of illnesses in a variety of clinical settings, and is essential to a well-rounded training program. The rotation of patients to settings that offer specialized technical care is considered essential to the provision of optimal medical treatment. Yet, perhaps to a greater extent than any other facet of the hospital's operation, rotation compromises the doctor–patient relationship.

Patient Rotations

It is not uncommon for a patient who is admitted to the hospital for chest pain to be transferred three, four, or even five times in the course of his hospital stay.

> Mr. T. was admitted from the emergency room to a medical ward for chest pain and questionable EKG abnormalities. Twenty-four hours later, he was transferred to the coronary care unit with an evolving myocardial infarction. After three days in the coronary care unit, he was moved to the intermediate coronary care unit for close but less intensive observation. Four days later he was transferred back to a medical ward, but not the one to which he had been admitted. One week later, the patient had stabilized. Accordingly, he was transferred, for the fifth time, to the self-care rehabilitation unit in preparation for discharge.

The prime consideration, of course, was to offer Mr. T. the best technical care available. But the fact that he was transferred to five different settings in the course of his hospital stay meant that he was cared for by as many residents and interns. Furthermore, he was ministered to by fifteen different shifts of nurses, three each per hospital unit.

House Staff Rotations

Even when the patient remains stationary, that is, on the same ward, there is no certainty that he will be treated by the same physician throughout his hospital stay. Apart from the value of house staff rotations for training purposes, such rotations are justified on humane grounds. Administration and staff share the view that residents and interns cannot be exposed around the clock, for a prolonged period, to the stresses of life on a busy medical ward.

> "It isn't that the care of patients itself is so difficult," said a bleary-eyed intern who had been up all night. "It's the struggle to get the routine things done—an X-ray, a hospital chart, an addressograph plate, a call through to the private doctor—that wears me out. And tomorrow I'll struggle with the same old things until I'm finally off this ward."

Nurse Rotations

As a rule, the nurse remains on the same ward. However, she may be rotated to different patients on that ward, to increase her exposure to a variety of clinical illnesses, and, at times, to ensure her physical and emotional survival.

> Mrs. Y., a 58-year-old beautiful and talented woman, whom the staff perceived as a warm, giving person, was dying of cancer. She had skin metastases, and her badly ulcerated left breast required pressure dressings. She stirred up such distress that her nurses had to rotate daily.

A nurse might also rotate if she were unable to tolerate the disruptive behavior of a problem patient. But rotation as a solution to the problem patient only makes the patient more of a problem—because continuing meaningful contact, the one therapeutic lever that has consistently proven helpful in the management of such patients, is no longer available.

The Rotation of Ward Attendings

The usual monthly rotation of ward teaching attendings is considered essential for two reasons. First, the house staff is thereby exposed to different clinical viewpoints, which enhances the training experience. Second, the attendings would find it a hardship to be involved with the ward for an extended period of time. During an attending's one-month tour of duty on a medical ward, for example, he must assume primary responsibility for forty patients, and the supervision of house officers and medical students. Moreover, during this period he must continue to fulfill his extramural professional responsibilities. It is not surprising, in light of this hectic and exhausting schedule, that proposals to extend the period of the attending's stay on the ward have met with resistance. But the fact that the attending's consequent limited contact with the ward population is justified on realistic grounds does not alter its adverse effects on both patients and staff.

The rotation of the house staff and ward attendings has a direct—and disastrous—effect on the operation and ambience of the ward. For example, in accordance with current administrative policy, the Chief of Medicine and his assistant are responsible for the overall management of six medical wards, all of which are as large as some individual services, such as neurology, oncology, pediatrics, and adolescence, and much larger than the single wards maintained by some specialties that constitute independent administrative entities, such as the intensive care unit (fourteen beds), the coronary care unit (ten beds), and the Department of Psychiatry (twenty-two beds). Obviously, the Chief of Medicine and his assistant cannot provide close surveillance of each of these six units, and no provision is made for the permanent assignment to the medical service of a physician who would be responsible for day-to-day management of these units. Consequently, responsibility for the operation of each unit falls, by default, to a rotating staff, whose commitment to the administrative operation of the ward is tenuous, and who are unlikely, therefore, to make any significant effort to improve the quality of medical or nursing care, or to effect long-term solutions to the routine problems that impede the efficient delivery of clinical services. In essence, the problem lies in the fact that the ward doesn't constitute an enduring cohesive unit.

THE PATIENT POPULATION

The hospital's patient population is divided into two major categories: private patients and staff patients. Patients in both these categories may, in addition to their private or staff patient status, be categorized as referred patients.

Private versus Staff-Patient Status

In recent years the extension of third-party coverage systems to larger segments of the population has produced a predictable steady increase in the number of private patients. Today, two-thirds of the medical patients and four-fifths of the surgical patients at Montefiore are private patients. Some institutions admit only staff patients; however, the majority of institutions admit both private and staff patients. Private patients are segregated at some institutions; at others, Montefiore among them, private and staff patients occupy the same rooms. In either event, there are two kinds of patients, and two kinds of care.

In contrast to the staff patient, who is treated by the house doctor to whom he has been assigned, the private patient is admitted to the hospital and "treated" by his own physician, with the tacit understanding that the private physician will provide a teaching experience for the house staff, in exchange for the privilege of using the hospital's facilities. However, the house staff do not always feel the trade-off is equitable.

Ideally, the private physician would fulfill his commitment to the hospital by demonstrating the value of the doctor–patient relationship for the edification of the house staff; moreover, by sharing his knowledge of the patient's prehospital life, and his plans for the patient's in-hospital and posthospital care with the staff, he can extend their understanding of the etiology and pathogenesis of disease. In actuality, however, the private patient is "off limits," in a sense, to the house staff. Although house doctors are expected to provide "body care" for these patients, as a general rule they do not collaborate with the private physician in formulating a treatment plan for his patient; and, in fact, the private physician often warns the house staff not to try to explore his patient's emotional life. It is not surprising, therefore, that the house staff feel the exchange is unbalanced and regard caring for the private patient as a chore or a technical exercise.

The Referred Patient

Teaching hospitals are centers of training, research, and clinical expertise in a variety of specialties. Consequently, a significant number of patients are referred to such institutions for diagnosis, evaluation, and treatment, with the understanding that they will return to their referring physician for follow-up care. However, the referred status is not reserved for patients who have been referred to the teaching hospital by their private physician. Even a patient who is "referred" to the inpatient service by a doctor from the hospital's ambulatory clinic is not cared for in the hospital by the doctor who made the referral. And, similarly, the inpatient doctor does not usually provide follow-up care for the patient after he has been discharged.

There is another category of referred patients: "referred-referred" patients. This category comprises those patients, many of whom are acutely ill, who are referred by their internist to a specialist—a neurologist or surgeon, for example—who, in turn, refers them to the hospital's neurological or surgical service for evaluation. The house officer on these wards thus is twice removed from the primary physician.

Apart from the fact that the house doctor may not be alert to the patient's adverse psychological reactions to his illness, or competent to manage these reactions in any event, the patient's referred status is sufficient, in itself, to disrupt the house doctor's holistic thinking, and foster mind–body dualism: many psychological issues can only be understood and treated in the context of an ongoing relationship. The referred patient is unknown to the house staff before his arrival at the hospital, and will not be seen again after he has been discharged. Consequently, the house doctor tends to concentrate on the patient's physical symptoms, and psychological issues (including the doctor–patient relationship) do not enter his thinking.

THE STAFF

The Clinical Staff

This section describes the psychological climate on the various clinical services at Montefiore, which, inevitably, reflects the attitudes toward psychological care of the senior and house staffs of that service.

The Surgical Service. Twenty-five percent of the patients who are hospitalized at Montefiore are admitted to the surgical service, which encompasses several wards under one administrative head. Many of these patients are emergency admissions, and have referred or referred-referred status. As is true of the medical service, no one senior person is present enough of the time to supervise the overall operation of a given unit. Moreover, the resultant deficits in the quality of psychological care are compounded by the fact that, in contrast to the internist, the surgeon spends a great deal of time off the ward, and away from his patients. By and large, the nurse is left in charge, but she is not given sufficient authority to take appropriate action if she identifies psychological dysfunctions.

When we reviewed the surgeons' requests for psychiatric consultation, we were impressed that there were so few; that requests for consultation were often received late in the course of the patient's hospitalization, when plans for his discharge were under way; and that, in many cases, psychiatric recommendations had not been put into effect. In addition, in many instances the surgeon who had requested the consultation had been in the operating room, and was not available to discuss the patient before or after he was seen by the psychiatrist.

We hypothesized that either the surgeon does not recognize psychological dysfunction, or believes that in most cases it lies within the range of normal preoperative or postoperative behavior. Therefore, he expects the patient (and the staff) to tolerate considerable emotional stress and distress.

The Medical Service.* The volume of consultations, of the reported incidence of depression or anxiety on one service, as opposed to another, may reflect staff attitudes toward these affects (and, by implication, toward the psychological needs of their patients). The largest number of requests for psychiatric consultation comes from the medical service, and they often include questions relating to differential diagnosis or management, which

* The structure and organization of the medical service were described earlier in this chapter.

presupposes a high level of psychological sophistication. And, in fact, many internists recognize that a significant number of their patients suffer from preexisting psychological difficulties that may complicate the management of their physical illness, and that an equal number of "normal" patients will manifest adverse psychological reactions to their medical illness.

The Oncology Service. The oncology service is run primarily by attendings, who are assisted in the day-to-day operation of the ward by the medical house staff who rotate monthly. Patient-staff relationships reflect the firm conviction that the terminally ill cancer patient should not be informed of either his diagnosis or prognosis. Consequently, conversation is kept to a minimum, so that the patient will not have an opportunity to ask questions. As a further precaution, the psychiatrist is asked "not to stir the patients up," for in that event they might press the physicians and nurses to tell them what is happening.

The monthly rotation of house staff, the brief visits of the attending, and the mandate not to talk combine to reduce the amount of meaningful psychological help afforded these patients. Fear, anxiety, feelings of abandonment and isolation are suppressed or alleviated by medication. More precisely, psychological "comfort" is provided via the widespread and liberal use of narcotics and hypnotics.

The Neurology Service. Basically, the neurology service, which consists of one ward under a single administrator, is concerned with diagnosis and teaching. Most of the patients on its busy, frequently overcrowded unit have been referred by their own internists, by the hospital's ambulatory clinics, or by their own neurologists for diagnosis of potentially life-threatening symptoms, and the great majority are emergency admissions. Diagnosis and treatment of the acute problem, then, is the first order of business. The focus of the house staff and the orientation of their teachers preclude meaningful concurrent consideration of the anatomical and psychological aspects of neurological illness.

The Faculty

Broadly stated, the training program at Montefiore has two overriding goals: to equip the student with the diagnostic and therapeutic skills that are basic to the practice of medicine, and to foster the holistic approach to patient care, which is the cardinal criterion of clinical competence. The content and orientation of the training program are at variance with these goals because of its emphasis on physiological considerations, and because the staff responsible for the implementation of this clinically oriented training program may not, themselves, be primarily involved with patient care. It is an unfortunate paradox that the reputation of the teaching hospital rests on the academic and research standing of its chiefs of service.

The fact that the prestigious role model may not be primarily involved in patient care constitutes a major source of conflict for the young house doctor whose primary professional goal is to treat patients. He may also be impeded in forming his professional identity by coming into contact with ward attendings who, although they are enaged in clinical practice, are nonetheless indifferent to their patients' psychological needs. Similarly, although they are engaged in training new doctors, they may be indifferent to their students' psychological needs, and focus instead on the technical aspects of medical practice.

> An abashed resident admitted he hated to examine a patient with massive edematous legs and stasis ulcers, and said he wondered how the patient must feel. The attending who was present at the time responded to what was obviously a request by the resident for help in managing his own feelings and dealing with the patient by asking him whether he knew where filaria was endemic in the Western Hemisphere. He then added that the resident should know the answer to this question because it was frequently asked on the Boards.

The apparent lack of interest of some role models and teachers in the mental life of patients and trainees has predictable consequences for their students. They learn that to be a good student, one does not talk about a patient's feelings or reactions (or about one's own feelings or reactions), but about electrocardiographic tracings, blood gases, medications, and host, vector, and infectious agents. The point is that these teachers, consciously or unconsciously, stymie the house doctor's efforts to understand his patient's psychological reactions as well as his own, and to expand his repertoire to include the knowledge, techniques, and self-awareness that will enable him to deal effectively with such reactions.

Other role models provide invaluable learning experiences for the house doctor.

> Mr. O., who was 78 years old, had been in the hospital for six months. He had chronic obstructive pulmonary emphysema and peripheral vascular disease, secondary to diabetes. His left leg had been amputated, and the stump required surgical revision for the attachment of a prosthesis. The patient was understandably despondent about the prospect of additional surgery, particularly because this would further prolong his separation from his 75-year-old wife, who journeyed some distance every day to visit.

The attending questioned the advisability of subjecting this patient to another surgical procedure. He felt that it was not realistic to expect Mr. O. to be able to use a prosthesis. Moreover, their prolonged separation was devastating to both the patient and his wife. The attending argued vigorously that the house doctor should terminate Mr. O.'s chronic hospitalization, which he felt was in pursuit of the doctor's need to reconstitute the patient, and not in accord with the realities of the patient's life situation.

By urging the student to view the patient holistically, and by helping him to become aware of his own feelings, this role model enabled him to gain a perspective that took into account the patient's psychosocial as well as his physical needs.

The Nursing Staff. Just as the doctor's role vis-à-vis his patient has changed since the days of St. Bernard, the function of the nurse and the quality of her relationship with the patient have changed radically since the time of Florence Nightingale.

In the contemporary teaching hospital, which epitomizes the social and technical revolution in medicine, the nurse on a busy medical ward does not provide primary nursing care in the strict sense of the term.* To begin with, no one nurse provides total nursing care for the patient. One nurse takes temperatures, another passes medication, a third charts orders; the patient may be admitted by still another nurse, who will be replaced by someone else the next day. As mentioned earlier, on some wards nurses may be assigned to take care of different patients every day. Nurses change shifts every eight hours. Moreover, at Montefiore the turnover in nursing personnel on a given ward may reach 30 percent in one year.†

The nurse's responsibility for the patient's psychological care varies on each service: Where the house staff is unavailable or unconcerned with the patient's psychological care, responsibility for such care falls to the nurse. Unfortunately, on the neurological, surgical, and oncology wards, where this situation prevails in particular, the nurse is not given the authority to ask for the psychiatric help she needs to perform this function.

The Social Service Staff. Social service is built into the structure of the ward in the teaching hospital; like other components of the system, it con-

---

* It should be noted, however, that this change in the nurse's role is unique to the teaching hospital. In small community hospitals, nurses run the wards; their presence on the ward remains constant; and they exert a fair amount of authority over the patient's milieu.
† This turnover rate refers to nurses who rotate within Montefiore, as well as to those who leave the hospital. Certain placements, on the intensive care and coronary care units, for example, are highly coveted, primarily because the nurses on these units exercise significant authority, almost commensurate with that of the house staff.

stitutes an autonomous unit, headed by its own director, with clearly defined precepts and goals. Unlike their colleagues on the ward, however, social workers are not viewed as members of the team.

This is unfortunate because the social worker is trained to evaluate the patient's psychological functioning, the quality of his family relationships, and his psychological environment outside the hospital. And, given this knowledge, plus the fact that she is based on the ward, she is in a unique position to detect adverse psychological reactions to medical illness; to understand the meaning of these reactions, and to make important recommendations as to how the patient's psychological and social needs can best be met while he is in the hospital and after he has been discharged.

In fact, however, the social worker is rarely given an opportunity to demonstrate her considerable expertise in this area. Instead, she is expected to perform what might be described as a housekeeping function. Specifically, the social worker is expected to talk with the patient's family or, when necessary, to tap community resources to procure concrete services on the patient's behalf. Furthermore, over the years, social workers have come to accept their professional fate. They assume responsibility for a limited "part of the action," as it were—at the physician's discretion. Having made his referral, the physician feels he no longer has to be concerned with this aspect of the patient's welfare. Thus, all too frequently, the social worker's efforts become an exercise in mind-body dualism.

The Patient Advocate. When a subcommittee of the Women's Auxiliary of Montefiore approached the Chief of Medicine to discuss ways in which they might provide more direct help for patients in the hospital, the decision was made to assign two women to a forty-bed medical ward on a trial basis. The patient advocates would be available daily to talk with individual patients and to elicit concrete requests for help. It was anticipated that their efforts might include arranging to rent a television set, requesting a family member to visit, helping a patient to feed himself, or asking the patient's physician or a nurse to see him in order to allay his anxiety. It was hoped that by bringing the patient's plight to the administration and by performing these relatively routine tasks, the patient advocates would gratify needs that were important to the patient, but that his physician, nurse, and social worker had neither the time nor the inclination to deal with. Thus they would highlight and at times fill the gap in patient services caused by the technological revolution in medicine.

The contention by both the medical service and the hospital administration that the patient needed an advocate cannot be disputed. But their decision to act on this realization meant that still another person was added to the corps of "piece workers" whose efforts were limited to the patient's humanistic needs that were, in fact, neglected by the overburdened physician and nurse. But in many cases the advocate was not qualified to evaluate the meaning of psychological distress in a patient—or, for that matter, to detect its presence.

For example, the advocate would frequently transmit a patient's request that the food be improved, or that his doctor come to examine him, or that the nurse answer his ring more promptly—which only increased the pressures on his caretakers and their feelings of guilt, but missed the point of why the patient had complained in the first place. The patient who is angry with the world because he was "chosen" to be a victim of a chronic disease, or who is apprehensive about his diagnosis, may—and often does—displace his anger and anxiety onto the house staff or the establishment. He will then try to justify his behavior on the grounds that the food is bad, the nurses inefficient, the doctors incompetent, and so forth. When the advocate remains oblivious to the patient's real complaint, she only increases his frustration—and perpetuates his dissatisfaction.

With the introduction of the patient advocate, the contemporary teaching hospital had come full circle. After subdividing the patient into a body, a mind, and a human being, it had recognized the dangers of leaving any one part unattended and had attempted to guard against such dangers by providing a caretaker for each subdivision. But no one caretaker had final responsibility for the patient as an entity.

THE PSYCHIATRIC WARD AS A PARADIGM OF
THE TEAM APPROACH TO PATIENT CARE

The organization of the psychiatric inpatient service at Montefiore Hospital can offer practical guidelines for the improvement of patient care on the hospital's medical and surgical wards. First, the ward is organized to ensure the development of viable patient–staff relationships and continuity of care. Primary care is provided by the psychiatric resident, nurse, and social worker who are assigned to a given patient throughout his hospitalization. When the patient is discharged from the inpatient service, the same psychiatric resident is expected to continue to treat him in the ambulatory clinic. Furthermore, if the patient is rehospitalized within the year, he will be admitted and treated by the same doctor.

Second, overall operation of the ward is supervised by a psychiatrist administrator, who is on the unit for several hours every day throughout the academic year, and who has primary responsibility for the quality of patient care, intrastaff relationships, and standards of training. At the same time, he is expected to improve the overall functioning of the unit and to develop new procedures that will enhance patient care (and enrich the training experience). In addition, dealing with routine problems is an important part of his job. His ability to "take the squeak out of the machinery" leaves the staff free to perform their essential caretaking functions.

Third, as mentioned above, the same nurse is assigned to a given patient throughout his hospitalization, and during this time she participates actively in the resident's diagnostic and therapeutic efforts. Thus, in contrast to other services, a unique relationship exists between the resident and the nurse. And the fact that they will work together for several months, and often throughout the entire academic year, strengthens that relationship. Inevitably, staff differences occur from time to time. However, they are mediated by the ward administrator, and are aired constructively. The nurse knows that her observations of the patient's behavior are an important source of information not only for her colleagues on the nursing staff while she is off duty, but for the entire staff; therefore, she records relevant data concerning the patient with the anticipation that her notes will be read.

Fourth, the psychiatric resident differs from residents in other specialties in several important respects. He remains on the ward for an entire year, and adapts to a milieu in which he is only one member of a team that provides comprehensive psychiatric care for the ward population. Furthermore, because the psychiatric resident frequently comes to the ward directly from medical school, it is openly acknowledged that he may be the least experienced member of the team; consequently, he does not enjoy special status on the ward, and finds it easier to ask for help. Thus, the usual doctor–boss, nurse–slave orientation is appropriately tempered.

More important, from the outset, the psychiatric resident is made aware of the fact that in-hospital care is essentially secondary prevention, and that acute psychiatric illness constitutes only one phase of the larger health–illness cycle he must master. Accordingly, evaluation of the patient during hospitalization includes consideration of primary prevention issues, that is, identification of the factors that precipitated his illness, and tertiary prevention issues, that is, continuity of care as a means of minimizing the possibility of relapse.

The social worker, who is an integral part of the team, may perform at all three levels. The social worker is concerned, in particular, with the quality of the patient's interpersonal relationships, and she stresses the importance of including an evaluation of this aspect of human behavior in every patient's work-up. In many instances, it is apparent that the nurse, resident, or social worker could care for the patient's psychological needs; in others, it is felt that the nurse or social worker might be more effective than the resident. When many patients are exposed to the team approach over a sufficiently long period of time, guidelines emerge with respect to the division of labor.

It is evident from our description of the psychiatric ward that major benefits accrue from a cohesive and closely supervised ward–unit system. The reorganization of medical and surgical wards so that they, too, might function as well-supervised cohesive units would require the implementation of administrative measures that would radically alter time-honored practices and relationships. In fact, such changes are in progress. The hospital is moving—slowly, but inexorably—from the advisory bureaucratic model (the "comb" effect) to an industrial bureaucratic model (the "tree" effect).* An industrial bureaucratic model would permit a powerful, centralized governing body without any particular territorial imperative. Such a governing body could ensure a cohesive unit in which conflicts between patient care, training, and research could be mediated more effectively, and which, therefore, would in itself provide a modicum of psychological well-being for the hospital's patient population.

* The formation of a union by interns and residents and their recent, and successful, use of a strike—the traditional tool of labor—against management are evidence of the move toward the industrial bureaucratic model in the contemporary teaching hospital.

Chapter 14

Building the Alliance

James J. Strain

Based on his understanding of the flaws in the operation of the teaching hospital, the liaison psychiatrist employs a two-pronged approach to achieve his goal. First, using his knowledge of the anatomy of the teaching hospital, he attempts to foster structural changes in the organization and operation of the patient care system whenever possible. Second, since the system is only as good as the people who run it, he uses the device of the teaching conference to reach the persons within the system who care for medical and surgical patients. Obviously, these strategies have a reciprocal effect. Structural changes in the system create a suitable milieu for the liaison psychiatrist's efforts to transmit data concerning the psychological care of the medically ill to the hospital staff. Innovative teaching conferences facilitate his efforts to make structural changes in the organization and operation of the wards.

In the advisory bureaucratic system, the liaison psychiatrist attempts to enlist the collaboration of the Department of Medicine, the Department of Nursing, the Department of Social Service, the Department of Psychiatry, and, finally, the hospital administration, in order to foster a holistic approach to patient care. In his efforts to build alliances with these departments, the liaison psychiatrist must assume a role that differs from the traditional role of the psychiatrist. In contrast to the consulting psychiatrist, who appears in response to a request for his services, the liaison psychiatrist must persuade the hospital administration and the heads of various departments of the importance of his services—of the importance of caring not only *for* the patient, but *about* the patient. This time-consuming and difficult task requires a measure of political expertise. More important, it requires the ability to work through others, rather than the self, and to press forward, often in the face of considerable resistance, which attacks one's narcissism, professional identity, and purpose.

EFFECTING STRUCTURAL CHANGE

Liaison psychiatry strives to effect structural changes in various departments throughout the hospital that will endure beyond the tenure of a given individual. For example, after it became apparent that psychological factors were responsible for the failure to maintain patients in the "life island" (the complete isolation technique) for immunosuppressant therapy of leukemia and aplastic anemia reactions, psychiatric clearance became mandatory for all life island candidates. Similarly, psychiatric clearance is now mandatory for all drug overdose patients before they are discharged from the intensive care unit. The point is that structural changes should become part of hospital routine, and not be dependent on the whim of a medical attending or a liaison psychiatrist. If nurses were empowered to request psychiatric consultation, neither the constant rotation of house staff nor a recalcitrant attending would negate the acquisition of appropriate psychiatric assistance. And if a department of medicine installed physician-administrators (ombudsmen) on each ward to monitor patient–staff and intrastaff issues, the constant presence of a liaison psychiatrist would not be necessary to foster psychological accountability.

For the liaison psychiatrist, building alliances depends on mutual trust, patience, and respect. Only then will he be privy to departmental issues that are normally kept from "outsiders." The liaison psychiatrist effects structural changes in the operation of these departments by offering suggestions, based on his observations, that are designed to promote "psychological-mindedness." It is hoped that as a result of these structural changes, psychological issues will be "in the air," and that they will become not only an intrinsic part of ward life and thinking, but of the overall operation of the hospital. To illustrate, if a brief mental screening device for medical patients were incorporated into every admission work-up, the physician would be forced to think about the possibility of organicity. Furthermore, high standards of patient care would be assured if, when the screening device reflected a certain minimal rating score, suggesting the possibility of organicity, the admitting physician would automatically request a psychiatric consultation, similar to the hematology consult that follows any hematocrit value below 30 mg/percent in our hospital. In addition, the use of techniques to assess mood disturbances (anxiety, depression) and maladaptive coping in the medically ill, and to counteract the inappropriate use of psychotropic drugs should be made part of hospital procedure.

The liaison psychiatrist makes a judgment as to what to do, where to do it, and with whom. Some services and wards do best with consultations; the house staff on these services are simply not interested in, or capable of, fulfilling the psychological needs of their patients. When a service is responsive to the concept of the team approach, the liaison psychiatrist enters into a "contract" with that service that is written to change the "guest in the house" status normally afforded the consulting psychiatrist to that of a bona fide member of the team. The contract includes a provisional clause: "I [the liaison psychiatrist] will show you how to provide psychological care for the patient, if you will agree to try to take over this function yourselves ultimately."

In summary, structural changes in patient care systems are presently brought about by the following: the liaison psychiatrist's ability to identify and work with chiefs of departments who are sympathetic to psychological issues, the concomitant development of appropriate role models, direct involvement of the physician and nurse in the psychological care of the patient, when possible, and a persistent liaison presence.

THE DYNAMICS OF THE TEACHING CONFERENCE

The second aspect of the two-pronged liaison approach is the innovative teaching conference. We proceed on the premise that the liaison teaching conference can create a situation in which feelings, ideas, misconceptions, fantasies, and inhibitions—which would otherwise remain undetected by the attendings and house staff—emerge. In this respect, it may be likened to the psychoanalytic situation that allows the analyst and the patient to view aspects of mental life that are usually hidden. Or it can be compared to the surgical situation that permits the surgeon to explore and examine anatomical structures ordinarily not seen. The histologist, biochemist, immunologist, and radiologist create ingenious situations that enable them to probe behind the scenes, heighten contrast, observe dynamic states, and see forces at work that then dictate the nature and scope of their activities. Similarly, the emergence in the liaison teaching conference of the forces that underlie psychological problems in patients and staff alike highlights the structural-administrative changes that are needed in patient care and teaching.

It takes courage on the part of the psychiatrist and the hospital staff to create the liaison situation. Neither the psychiatrist nor the medical staff can be certain in advance of what they will learn. However, the material that arises is explored in a controlled, beneficial way. At the outset, the liaison psychiatrist establishes the fact that it is not his intention to provide the staff with a group therapy experience or a course in psychopathology; nor will he attempt to impose his moral or ethical values on them. At the same time, he assures them that any disclosures they may make in the course of the conference with regard to their professional attitudes and behavior, their response to a particular patient, or their feelings about the system will not be held against them. Nevertheless, creation of and participation in the liaison situation require skill, tact, maturity, and a spirit of inquiry.

THE DEPARTMENT OF MEDICINE

The Department of Medicine at Montefiore Hospital and Medical Center has a traditional interest in the holistic approach to patient care, dating back to the time when the hospital was a chronic disease center and emphasized the humane treatment of patients who could be offered little else in the way of medical care. This attitude persists today. Over the past five years, the Chief of Medicine has had an excellent relationship with the Department of Psychiatry, and has used its consultation services more frequently than has any other department in the hospital.*

When we initiated our program, the Department of Medicine responded favorably to our request that second-year residents in psychiatry be given liaison training on the medical wards. Accordingly, one resident was assigned to each of the six 40-bed medical units that comprise that service. They spent ten to twelve hours a week seeing patients, making rounds, and chairing separate weekly conferences for physicians and nurses, under the supervision of attending psychiatrists experienced in liaison procedures. By and large, these second-year residents felt overwhelmed by the responsibility that had been conferred on them, and they were uncomfortable in their role as specialty consultants in charge of a liaison program. Other specialty service consultants were chief residents. Most specialty teaching was done by junior attendings. Time after time, one or another liaison psychiatric resident had to report that he had been unable to round up the house staff for his conference. Their supervisors found that they no longer functioned as such: Instead, their efforts centered on the repair of hurt feelings, and on helping the resident to plan a strategy whereby he could persuade the house staff to give up an hour for a "psych conference." It was obvious that in order to counteract that pejorative label, a more senior person from the Department of Psychiatry was needed to head the liaison conference, and the conference had to be identified as an integral part of medical training.

Once the issues involved were clearly understood, a liaison fellowship was created that placed junior attending psychiatrists on three medical wards. The Department of Medicine agreed to make attendance at weekly conferences on the psychological aspects of patient care mandatory for the house staff. To further impress the house staff with the importance of

* This program evolved in collaboration with David Hamerman, Chief of Medicine, Montefiore Hospital and Medical Center.

psychological issues, the conferences on the three liaison wards, which were part of medical attending rounds, were co-chaired by the monthly medical attendings, who were selected on the basis of psychological aptitude, interest, and their capacity as role models to promote the holistic approach. Data were transmitted at the conference through discussion of the psychological evaluation, diagnosis, and management of medical patients, as well as discussion of the effects of medical illness on personality and behavior. Psychopharmacological issues, psychological treatment techniques, and countertransference responses to behavior were considered in terms of specific problem patients who were interviewed at the conference by their own house doctor.

At this point, psychological interviewing, evaluation, diagnosis, and the management of the medically ill were done by the medical doctor, on Medicine's time, under the tutelage of the medical attending, with the liaison psychiatrist serving as resource specialist. The medical attending's tutelage was not entirely satisfactory, however. The central problems were the monthly medical attending rotation system and the limited time the attending could spend on the ward, which restricted his involvement in the day-to-day operation of the ward, his supervision of the care of private patients, and his ability to modify house staff attitudes or perspective.

In contrast, the liaison psychiatric attending was on the medical ward every day throughout the academic year. He was aware of the day-to-day problems that arose on the ward; he knew the staff and the patients, and was, therefore, in an ideal position to affect the organization and administration of the ward. But the liaison psychiatrist did not have the authority to intervene in matters relating to the medical care of the patients and the operation of the ward. What was needed was the constant presence of a "medicine man" who would be responsible for the medical and psychological care provided on the ward, and who could teach the attitudes and perspective that are essential to a holistic view of the patient's needs.

When this was brought to the attention of the Chief of Medicine, he agreed to assign a medical ombudsman to each of the three liaison wards on a permanent basis. Specifically, the ombudsmen would be present on the wards daily for an entire academic year, and would meet weekly with their house staff, the liaison fellow, the ward social worker, and the nursing supervisor to handle major intrastaff and patient–staff conflicts. We envisioned these three liaison wards as "islands of excellence": Medicine, Nursing, Social Service, and Psychiatry would be sufficiently available to establish a milieu where physiological, psychological, and social issues existed in an interreacting matrix.

It was to our advantage that the Chief of Medicine and his assistant director agreed to serve as ombudsmen on two of the wards, and that the third ombudsman had a special interest in psychosocial issues and medical training. We hoped that by working with their house staff in this unique way, the Chief of Medicine and his assistant director would become aware of issues ordinarily kept hidden by the system—the problems posed by the increase in patient admissions, the private patient–staff conflict, the anxiety and sense of abandonment felt by the house staff, and the lack of attention given to the psychological perspective of the developing physician.

The Teaching Conference

The weekly liaison teaching conferences were structured to permit these issues to emerge.

At one such conference, a medical resident, Dr. T., attempted to interview a private patient she had been assigned to, who had been hospitalized for hypertension. When Dr. T. tried to talk to Mr. M., he said he was not her patient, and would only listen to his "real doctor," Dr. K. (Mr. M.'s private physician, who had been too busy to attend the conference).

After Mr. M. left the conference, Dr. T. expressed her feelings about the situation.

DR. T.: I really am annoyed with Dr. K. I don't agree with his treatment approach, and he won't discuss it with me. It seems to me that a treatment plan that includes salt loading for a hypertensive patient is a little bizarre. I'm angry with Mr. M. too, and I'm ashamed of my attitude. I feel I've been neglecting him. Because I feel hostile toward Mr. M., I avoid him at morning rounds.

OMBUDSMAN: I understand your dilemma. When a private physician isn't available to explain the rationale for his treatment, and the patient is as cantankerous as Mr. M., you really do have a problem.

Two weeks later, Dr. T. reported on Mr. M.'s current status.

DR. T.: Mr. M. had a cerebral vascular accident and a pulmonary embolus. He's comatose, and in the intensive care unit. I'm outraged that Dr. K. insisted that a patient with such massive impairment be resuscitated. I'm angry too because I was a part of the treatment plan that caused this catastrophe.

DR. L. (*another resident*): How do you determine who should be resuscitated? What are the criteria? What I mean is, how do you get on the list?

OMBUDSMAN (*to interns*): How do you feel about this?

DR. P. (*an intern*): I don't think I would know when I should decide to let a patient die. But the thing that bothers me even more is that even if I felt a patient should live, I might not be able to get optimal treatment for him. I have a patient now who's deteriorating with severe respiratory disease. I feel he should be helped, but there's no bed available for him on the pulmonary intensive care unit.

DR. T.: I had a terrible weekend. My mother-in-law died. But the night before she died, my husband and father-in-law—they're both doctors, you know—and I sat at her bedside. My mother-in-law had advanced cancer, and didn't want another hospitalization. I gave her pain medication to let her sleep, but one dose wasn't enough. [*Tearfully*] I just don't think it's right to resuscitate Dr. K.'s patient.

OMBUDSMAN (*with obvious feeling*): I just don't think we're giving you residents and internists the help you need. We're not making it easier for you to deal with private physicians, and we're not helping you to deal with the dying, the elderly, and with chronically ill patients.

This teaching conference was unique in several respects. The ombudsman (who was the Chief of Medicine) was made acutely aware of the problems of the house staff, and it was he, rather than the liaison psychiatrist, who verbalized these issues. At the same time, he was made acutely aware of the need for the medical attending to be more involved with the life of the ward—and more sensitive to the issues that had emerged at this conference but that "never cross the director's desk." Although it was not our intention to simulate a T-group, or to provide a psychotherapeutic experience for the staff, the conference was structured so that it would go beyond the routine aspects of patient care to encompass the feelings of the house staff. It is unlikely that current models of teaching would have allowed these issues to emerge. And it is just as unlikely that the house staff would have shared their strong personal feelings with each other off the ward. This teaching conference legitimized exploration by the staff of perspectives and feelings that were in conflict with traditional professional attitudes.

On another occasion, Dr. B., an intern, asked that Mrs. R., a 31-year-old woman who was dying of cancer, be interviewed and discussed at the teaching conference. Although the patient, who had two young children, was scheduled for discharge after the conference, Dr. B. felt she should be seen because "her behavior was bizarre." She had kissed him, asked if she could call him by his first name, and, at the same time, told him she had a malignancy. Mrs. R.'s private physician agreed that she could be presented, but the ombudsman was reluctant to have her seen at the conference. He felt it would be too stressful for the patient if the staff talked about cancer and dying in front of her. He agreed to have her presented only after the liaison fellow and her private physician had assured him it would be all right, and that it might even be helpful.

DR. B. (*to the patient*): Can you tell us what it's like to have a malignancy?

MRS. R.: I know I'm dying. I just hope I'll have a few more months to be with my daughters. They're so young. I'm worried about what other people may have told them about me. When I get home, they may be afraid to hug me; they may even be afraid to let me touch them. I feel like a Typhoid Mary. My children may think that if they come near me, they'll catch my disease.

LIAISON PSYCHIATRIST: You're the one who's afraid you're infectious, but you must know that your children can't catch your disease. You can touch them and hold them as much as you like. If you know for a fact that your mother-in-law or your neighbors have told your children not to go near you, you'll just have to set them straight.

At the end of the interview, Mrs. R. said it had been a great relief just to be able to talk to someone about cancer, and dying, and about her fear that her disease might be catching. She then got up, kissed the intern, thanked the staff for taking care of her, and said she hoped she wouldn't need them for a while. She turned next to her private physician, kissed him, and on her way out, in an aside to the group, said, "He isn't afraid to touch me. I guess I'm not as frightening or ugly as I thought, even though I do have cancer." After Mrs. R. left, the conference continued.

DR. F. (*resident*): I don't think it's right for patients to behave that way.

DR. S. (*resident*): Right. Limits should be set for such patients.

LIAISON PSYCHIATRIST: You've missed the point. If Mrs. R.'s doctor had rebuked her, she would have taken that as an omen that she would be rejected by her children; she would have interpreted his rebuke as proof that she was infectious and repulsive. Mrs. R. acted out because she needed some real reassurance—not just verbal reassurance—before she returned home.

The psychological stresses typically evoked in the doctors of dying patients—the anxiety because their inability to offer a cure, their fear of hurting the patient, making him angry, or disturbing what they assume must be a tenuous psychological balance—almost kept the ombudsman from permitting Mrs. R. to participate in this conference. As a result of the conference, there was a shift in his position. He recognized the value of this opportunity for physicians to learn how to talk to patients about death. Similarly, the house doctors who were in daily contact with such patients learned that they could ask them how they felt about having cancer, and even let themselves be kissed, if that meant fulfilling their apostolic function: to care for the patient's mind as well as his body.

A few months later, the liaison fellow on another medical ward was faced with the problem of how to approach a new intern (Dr. W.) who had repeatedly referred patients who made him angry for psychiatric consultation. He finally decided to ask the intern to present one of the patients he felt needed psychiatric help at a teaching conference. And, in effect, this young doctor helped us to help him by bringing his feelings and behavior out into the open in the liaison situation. Mrs. D., the patient presented, had been hospitalized for the third time with a serious heart condition, and was assertive, directive, and highly critical of the medical and nursing staff. Dr. W. felt she was petty, negative, uncooperative, and demanded "more than her share" of care.

DR. W. (*to patient*):   Do you feel it's fair to ask for so much help, especially since you're not that sick? I feel you're demanding and uncooperative. Do you realize that you make me very angry?

MRS. D.:   I'm very upset that you feel this way about me. I don't want to make you angry; my life depends on you. I'm afraid you may make a mistake, or that you won't be around when I need you, that you'll let me die. I'm afraid to be alone.

Mrs. D. left after this exchange and the conference continued.

OMBUDSMAN (*to Dr. W.*):   You have to learn to get some distance from a patient. You can't limit your practice to patients you like, and expect to make a living. What would you do if a patient wanted to seduce you? I think it's important that you learn to handle your own feelings, so that you can treat all kinds of patients. If you get angry with them, the game is over: you can't use your medical knowledge, and the patient can't be helped.

Later, the ombudsman told the liaison fellow that he felt this had been the best medical conference he had run in a long time. He recognized that it was essential to teach attitudes and perspective to the house staff, and again deplored the fact that somehow these issues got lost on medical rounds that traditionally focused on facts and diagnosis. Most important, the ombudsman realized that this intern was in trouble, and asked the liaison psychiatrist how the medical staff could help him. The liaison situation had brought teacher and student together, and put them to work on essential issues.

Comment. The weekly liaison conferences demonstrated vividly the value of the "island of excellence" experiment on the three medical wards, and thereby facilitated further structural changes in the department's operation. Specifically, the Chief of Medicine agreed to establish medical ombudsmen on all medical wards, with a shift in responsibility for psychological accountability from the liaison fellow to the medical ombudsman. The liaison fellow on each ward would reduce his half-time commitment, and the medical ombudsman would assume responsibility for the day-to-day operation of the ward. Thus, the goal of liaison psychiatry was achieved. After transmitting his knowledge and skills to the staff, the liaison psychiatrist withdrew to permit the members of the Department of Medicine to do the job themselves, although he continued to function as a resource person.

In summary, an important structural change has occurred in the operation of the medical wards: someone (the ombudsman) is "tending the ward"; moreover, that person subscribes to the view that psychological considerations are an important and continuing aspect of patient care.

Clearly, this represents a major advance. Unfortunately, however, at present the ombudsman cannot devote as much time to the ward as is required to ensure its efficient operation. The final step in the evolution of our efforts to build an alliance with the Department of Medicine will be to persuade the hospital administration to make sufficient funds available for placement of a half-time medical attending on each ward, who would provide continuing, day-to-day supervision of medical and psychological care.

AMBULATORY MEDICAL CARE SERVICES

As opposed to the busy medical wards, working in the ambulatory setting had many advantages for teaching the liaison approach to patient care.

1. The medical staff does not rotate in the outpatient service as often. Consequently, the liaison psychiatrist could work with the same group of house doctors throughout the academic year.
2. The patients selected for discussion by the house doctors were not referred patients but patients from their own rosters.
3. In the ambulatory setting one tends to see patients who are bothered more by their emotional reactions to medical illness than their illness per se.
4. Patients seen in the outpatient service are not usually involved in a life or death struggle (which, of course, would divert attention from psychological issues).

Two liaison teaching models were established in the ambulatory setting. First, liaison psychiatrists conducted weekly conferences for six to eight physicians from one of the folowing groups: (1) medical residents who had selected this teaching experience, (2) junior medical attendings, and (3) residents in social medicine (who are primary care physicians). A senior medical attending (ombudsman) participated in each conference, at which interviewing, evaluating, and core liaison issues were discussed around specific patients in the physicians' panels. The junior medical attendings, who ran the medical Outpatient Department, hoped, once they had acquired sufficient psychological knowledge and skills, to provide a liaison training experience for all internal medicine residents on the outpatient service. The group of residents in social medicine wanted to acquire knowledge and skills that would enable them to fulfill the psychological, as well as the medical, needs of the patients at a large medical health center (Martin Luther King, Jr., Health Center).

Second, a liaison modular unit consisting of a psychiatrist and a social worker was created to care for ambulatory renal dialysis and transplant patients, many of whom have significant psychological problems. It was not feasible to expect the psychiatric outpatient clinic, which was manned principally by residents who were not adequately trained in the psychology of the medically ill to assume responsibility for the care of over two hundred renal patients. In fact, it was generally recognized throughout the hospital that very few medical patients were considered eligible for treatment in the psychiatric outpatient clinic. Ultimately, we were able to solve this problem. Since most of the renal patients had federal or state medical assistance to pay for psychiatric care, we were able to serve this population by establishing a liaison team sustained by fees generated. In effect, we offered every renal dialysis and transplant patient psychological evaluation and treatment in the medical setting at minimum cost to the hospital. Because a considerable part of the cost of this service was defrayed by third-party payers, the hospital administration was able to authorize the renal dialysis liaison team. Otherwise, necessary budgetary constraints on new and existing programs would have prevented the addition of these essential psychiatric services.

The liaison modular unit offered twenty-five to thirty psychiatric hours per week. It was planned that when this unit was fully utilized, another modular unit would be added to serve the radiotherapy ambulatory clinic. Such stepwise development could continue through the other specialty and general medical clinics for at least one-third of the patients seen in these clinics who have federal or state medical coverage.

THE DEPARTMENT OF SOCIAL SERVICE

Social Service had a new director who was enthusiastic about the liaison approach.* Specifically, he hoped that social workers would be given more opportunity to provide psychological care for medical and surgical patients. As noted earlier, although social workers were available on the wards to serve as emotional caretakers, they were overwhelmed with disposition cases and were not an integral part of the health care team. The director also felt that the social worker should function as a teacher on the medical wards, and show physicians and nurses how to interview families.

Initially, the Departments of Social Service and Psychiatry had little meaningful exchange. Requests for consultation were received by both, with little indication of why the referring physician had selected one rather than the other to see the patient. At times, both services were called, and at times either could officiate. To get a better idea of each other's clinical capacities, all psychiatric consultations were answered for six weeks by both social service workers and liaison psychiatrists. Each patient was evaluated by both a social worker and a psychiatrist, and each service made up its mind independently as to who was better equipped to treat the patient. A high concordance was reached by the social workers and psychiatrists as to the disposition of these requests for consultation, that is, those best handled by the psychiatrist, the social worker, and those that required conjoint effort. However, the referring physicians oversubscribed to the use of the psychiatrist. Two-thirds of their requests could have gone to the social worker; only one-third should have gone exclusively to the psychiatrist. It was agreed that consultation requests needed to be audited, and that physicians needed further indoctrination in the use of social workers.

The idea of an "island of excellence"—a ward with a full-time social worker who was present at rounds and conferences, and who, as a member

---

* This program evolved in collaboration with Gerald Beallor, Director of the Department of Social Service, Montefiore Hospital and Medical Center.

of the liaison team, would educate physicians and nurses and, in turn, be educated by them—was appealing to the Social Service Department. Accordingly, the social worker became a member of a teaching conference in which she instructed the physician in what her abilities were and in the scope of her function with regard to patient care. She could influence history taking and conference presentation, and promote the use of family members in the management of the patient. Furthermore, she could move from patient referral to identifying those patients, from the total ward roster, who could benefit from the services of a social worker. In short, like the psychiatrist, she could shape attitudes and perspective, as well as elevate standards of patient care.

The struggle of the Department of Social Service and Psychiatry to find their identity on the medical ward occurred over a period of time, and underwent four developmental stages. At first, as indicated above, the two specialities worked as separate entities, with virtually no contact. During the second stage, each specialty became aware of the other, and contact was made, but they continued to work independently. At the third stage, the boundaries between the two services blurred: social workers and liaison psychiatrists worked side by side and "lumped" their efforts. In this phase there was little separation or individuation of function; much of the work was done conjointly. Unfortunately, however, efficiency fell, for conjoint efforts meant that the number of patients seen by the two services diminished significantly. As a general rule, the feeling of comfort produced by the lumping of activities and the consequent decreased patient coverage inhibit progress to the fourth stage and lead to abandonment of a more mature, differentiated working relationship for two reasons. First, the comfort of working together is a resistance to working independently and moving on. And, second, supervisors view the inefficiency of the team approach in the "lumping" phase as evidence that the experiment has failed. Customarily, the services involved then revert to a second- or first-phase relationship. In our experiment, we were able to "work through" these problems, with the result that Social Service and Psychiatry were able to move on to the fourth phase in their development. At this final stage, Social Service and Psychiatry operated independently, each with a sense of separate identity and a knowledge of the other that allowed for maximum individual effort and appropriate referral.

Ideally, in time Psychiatry and Social Service would have developed similar relationships with Medicine and Nursing on the "island of excellence" wards. The ultimate liaison achievement would be maximal autonomous functioning within each service and maximal appropriate use of the other's service. However, only Psychiatry and Social Service approached this fourth stage, presumably because they share a common purpose and orientation.

THE DEPARTMENT OF NURSING

Inasmuch as they are responsible for the day-to-day management of medical and surgical patients, nurses have firsthand knowledge of the consequences of a treatment approach that focuses exclusively on the patient's physical needs. It is not surprising, therefore, that from the outset the Director of Nursing was enthusiastic about the liaison approach.* Moreover, she was eager to cooperate in our efforts to make structural changes on the ward that would facilitate the formation of a more cohesive unit—to the extent that she was willing to give up a nursing position to make way for a lay administrator of the unit.

The Director of Nursing was concerned that within three months the humanistic ideals of a new nurse were usually eroded by the teaching hospital system. Unfortunately, our efforts to revitalize these ideals were similarly impeded by the system. Increased patient admissions, the fractionation of nursing duties, and the rotation of nurses on some services, which impeded the development of meaningful, continuing relationships with patients, also placed a serious limitation on liaison goals, especially nurses' continuing development and their move toward autonomy in regard to psychological care.

The liaison psychiatrist tailored his efforts to the kind of nursing practiced on a given service.

Surgery

The nurse's role on the surgery service was described in Chapter 10. The surgeons were very tolerant of anxious, even psychotic behavior, ascribing it to the not infrequent postoperative occurrences that subside with time and recovery. Meanwhile, the nurse had to care for delusional, hallucinating, anxious, depressed patients, and the patients simply had to live with their frightening, chaotic symptoms until they resolved spontaneously. It was not the liaison psychiatrist's or the nurse's expectation that the surgeon could or should be able to manage all the psychological needs of his patients. But it was their hope that he would at least permit the nurses to be the primary psychological caretakers if he could not assume that role himself. In fact, although they did not have the surgeon's official sanction, in his absence the nurses were the patient's primary caretakers. Thus our task was to provide them with training to fulfill this mission more adequately. We initiated three programs to this end.

* This program evolved in collaboration with Gale Kuhn, Former Director of Nursing, Montefiore Hospital and Medical Center.

1. At the request of the nurses, weekly meetings were held with the liaison psychiatrist on the most difficult surgery ward, the vascular ward, to examine nursing and patient problems. The nurses asked for help with their own feelings, and advice about management of the disruptive psychological reactions of their patients. The patients' adverse experiences with physicians and illness were often displaced onto the nurses, who were poorly equipped to handle such a massive assault on their personal and professional capacities. The nurses were distraught that, despite their best efforts, patients were still unhappy, and families continued to berate the staff about the miseries their loved ones had to endure. In an effort to alter this situation, a liaison psychiatrist met weekly with the nurses and weekly with the Chief of the Vascular Division; at the same time, a social worker led group meetings for patients to decompress their intense reactions. After three months the nurses and patients on the vascular ward and the social worker felt that tensions had been reduced.

2. At present, the liaison psychiatrist and a nurse from the psychiatric inpatient unit meet weekly throughout the academic year with the clinical nursing supervisors on the surgical service. Interviewing, psychological stress, and the core liaison problems discussed in Part II of this book are illustrated by pertinent clinical cases. More important, however, the nurses' "resistances" to learning about patients' emotional life are explored to enable them to take in and utilize psychological information heretofore isolated and intellectualized.

3. Nurses from our psychiatric inpatient unit with experience in the liaison setting are available to the surgical nursing staff for direct consultation. A request for a psychiatric nurse consultation bypasses the issue of obtaining the physician's permission to request a psychiatric consultation.

The structure has not been changed as yet to permit surgical nurses to initiate formal requests for psychiatric consultation in order for them to function more autonomously as the surgical patients' primary psychological caretakers.

Medicine

When the liaison program was initiated, and for two years thereafter, the Assistant Director of Nursing for medicine attended a weekly Medicine-Liaison luncheon with the Assistant Director of Medicine, the chief residents, liaison fellows, and the Director of the Liaison Service, at which physician–nursing issues, problem patients, the utilization and effectiveness of liaison intervention, and approaches to patient care were discussed.

At present, the liaison psychiatrist meets weekly with the Assistant Director of Nursing for medicine, and with all the clinical supervisory nurses on the medical service (just as he does with the supervisory nurses on the surgical service). It is our hope that enhancing the skills of this leadership group will have an optimal effect on the entire medical nursing staff.

A third attempt to establish a liaison program for nurses on the medical service involved the participation of psychiatric liaison nurses, who met with the nurses on the medical wards, without an assigned liaison attending. We wanted to evaluate the effects of psychiatrist-led versus nurse-led liaison units—to see if nurses should teach nurses. On one medical ward the psychiatric nurse was well received; on another, the medical nurses resented her presence. The efficacy of this technique as a vehicle for liaison teaching requires further study.

Finally, weekly Nursing-Liaison teaching conferences were held for several years on all medical wards.

The Teaching Conference. The Nursing-Liaison teaching conferences focused on interviewing and practical understanding of the patient's behavior, as illustrated below.

NURSE M.:   Mr. L. keeps wandering in and out of patients' rooms; female patients are especially bothered by his unannounced visits. He teases us too, and tries to touch us in a suggestive way. We try to avoid him as much as possible, I just hope he'll go home soon. This morning when I went into his room to take his vital signs, he pointed to a nude pinup at his bedside. Then he said, "How's that for a morning starter?" I got out of there as soon as I could.

The patient was then asked to join the teaching conference, and was interviewed by Nurse M.

NURSE M.:   How do you feel about your illness? Do you miss your family?

After several minutes of preliminary exploration.

LIAISON PSYCHIATRIST: How do you feel about Nurse M.?

MR. L.:   I don't know why I've been acting this way. Ever since my ulcer started to bleed, I've felt unsure of myself; I wonder how much of a man I am. I guess I'm trying to get a reaction out of them to see if I've got anything going for me. If only someone would tell me to stop, I think I'd feel I'm going to be alright. You don't take candy away from a baby who's going to die. Now, I know I'm not dying, but I don't know what's going on inside or where this blood is coming from. Maybe I had better get my kicks while I can.

The patient then left, and the conference continued.

LIAISON PSYCHIATRIST: By not setting limits on Mr. L.'s behavior, we've supported his fantasy that he is badly damaged.

NURSE M.: I was afraid I would hurt his feelings. It never occurred to me that he would interpret my failure to stop him as proof that he was very sick.

NURSE E.: I felt Mr. L. was disgusting. It was like having my father make a pass at me. It was embarrassing to take his blood pressure while he was pointing to that picture of the nude.

NURSE Q.: I've had more experience than you, and I wonder whether you felt you had to avoid him because he stimulated you.

NURSE M. (*to the liaison psychiatrist*): In other words, what you're trying to tell us is that Mr. L. isn't just a dirty old man. We've been hurting him and ourselves by not setting limits. I think I'll try to talk to him this week. I'll tell you how things work out.

Here is an excerpt from Nurse M.'s conversation with Mr. L.

NURSE M.: Mr. L., I know you're upset, but you just can't wander in and out of other patients' rooms.

MR. L. (*crying*): I guess I've been trying to get you gals as upset as I am. Here I want you to like me, and instead I drive you away.

The following week Nurse M. reported on her talk with Mr. L. at the teaching conference.

NURSE M.: Mr. L. told me how worried he was about regaining his health and apologized for being a bad boy. You know he's really a sensitive, decent guy. I think we had him pegged wrong. Incidentally, he's taken his nude pinup down.

Comment. The liaison situation made it possible for the nurses to view this patient in an entirely new light—and to examine their own feelings as well. They were able to see how their attitudes had contributed to inadequate nursing and to the patient's continuing despair. In the liaison situation, material heretofore hidden becomes manifest in a nondidactic fashion that permits its real acceptance. The nurses gradually learn to talk with their patients, to understand and manage difficult behavior, and they feel more secure as a result.

Oncology

After several years of liaison intervention and weekly teaching conferences, the preeminent characteristics of the oncology ward—the sanitized environment, the "resounding silence," and the narcotized patients —had changed dramatically. The nurses had breathed life back into the ward of the dying. Today, the ward is decorated with green plants and bright posters; patients are given hospital passes whenever possible; and they have become sufficiently involved in the world around them to stock and care for a fish tank. Most important, patients are encouraged to talk with their nurses.

To accomplish this, teaching conferences were held each week, and the nurses became increasingly concerned with how these patients' remaining months or days could be made more fulfilling. The liaison psychiatrist was able to heighten the nurses' awareness of the patient's clinical reaction to drugs; he taught them how to help patients adapt to their illness; and how to effect family interventions, so that the patient and his loved ones could remain close at a time when their need for closeness was greatest. Each week a patient was interviewed at the teaching conference, to demonstrate that approaching patients about their feelings could have a beneficial effect, and, in time, nurses became less frightened when patients asked: "Am I going to die?" "Will my husband love me with just one breast?" "Do I smell?" "Can I give my cancer to someone else if I touch them?" "Did this come from something I did?"

Neurology

Like the nurses on the surgical service, the nurses on the neurological service felt that the patients had been psychologically abandoned by their physicians, and wanted to provide such care on their own. They showed outstanding ability to absorb the basic data we transmitted on the psychology of the medically ill. Moreover, they learned to elicit the patients' fears and anxieties.

The Coronary Care Unit

The nurses in the coronary care unit asked for help with their own feelings. They found it difficult to talk with an acutely ill coronary patient because of their own anxiety that they might say something that would upset him. In addition, these highly trained nurses were always fearful that an inexperienced house officer might inadvertently endanger a patient's life. Nor were their relationships with their peers entirely satisfactory. Because they worked under constant tension, they were frequently irritable with each other.

Comment. Over the years the relationship between the nurses on these various services and the liaison psychiatrist has fluctuated. At times, it has been excellent; at other times, it has not fared as well. Nurses, like doctors, vary in their response to psychological data.

THE DEPARTMENT OF PSYCHIATRY

The liaison psychiatrist occupies a unique position, with one foot planted in the medical and surgical services and the other in the Department of Psychiatry.

Essentially, the Department of Psychiatry in a teaching hospital performs two functions. It offers a residency training program, and provides limited inpatient and outpatient facilities to serve the community and the hospital's medical and surgical population. An acutely psychotic patient from the medical or surgical division poses three problems for psychiatry. First, the patient who remains on the psychiatric ward for only a few days is an "intruder" in a milieu that focuses on ongoing psychotherapy. Second, the nursing and medical needs of the medical-psychiatric patient are often so urgent that they intrude on the psychiatric nurse's job to offer psychiatric help on the ward, or exceed the proficiency of the psychiatric nurse and psychiatric resident to adequately care for the patient's body, even with good medical backup. Third, the ward is usually full, so that admitting a psychotic medical patient means that one must go over census, or in some instances reluctantly arrange for the premature discharge of a psychiatric patient. On the other hand, to transfer the medically ill patient to another psychiatric facility would further enforce the mind–body dualism that currently characterizes our approach to patient care. In any event, the inability of the Department of Psychiatry's inpatient service to adequately care for the needs of the hospital's medical and surgical population undermines the liaison psychiatrist's efforts to effect alliances with the medical and nursing staff. Moreover, it may undermine his standing in the Department of Psychiatry as well. For the liaison psychiatrist is often placed in the uncomfortable position of siding with medicine against psychiatry.

The Department of Psychiatry also offers ambulatory diagnostic treatment facilities that serve the community and the hospital, and provide a resource for its training program. Traditionally, outpatient psychiatric care has been delivered by psychiatric residents. Since the number of patients they can see is limited, waiting lists get longer, and intake procedures become more selective to screen out those patients who are "least amenable" to treatment. By and large, this includes patients whose psychological dysfunction is a consequence of their medical illness. Residents treat only the psychosomatic or somatopsychic patients that they find particularly "interesting."

The problem is compounded by current administrative policies: medical clinics admit all patients, regardless of where they live, but the psychiatric clinic limits its admission to patients who live in the district or catchment area served by Montefiore. The Department of Psychiatry accepts a patient who lives outside the catchment area for treatment reluctantly and only if the hospital has a major medical obligation toward that patient.

These administrative policies tend to discourage the medical doctor from sending his psychologically disturbed patient for help if he doesn't live in the right catchment area. The liaison psychiatrist must make his department aware of the adverse side effects of these policies whether they are motivated by practical or training consideration. But, above all, he must serve as a model for his department. That is, he must be able to persuade his colleagues of the value and importance of psychological care for the medically ill, for only then can he hope to serve as a model for other departments throughout the hospital.

All psychiatric residents and fellows should have major instruction and training in the psychology of the medically ill. Often this can best be accomplished through the teaching conference.

The Teaching Conference

A 46-year-old married Puerto Rican woman who was a patient in Montefiore's Arthritis Clinic was asked to talk to a rheumatologist (Dr. V.), the psychiatric residents, and liaison fellows about her illness. According to her chart notes, Mrs. E. was a "chronic complainer." She was often tearful, felt that her illness was "unfair," and was extremely pessimistic about her future.

LIAISON PSYCHIATRIST: How are you feeling, Mrs. E.?

MRS. E. (*pointing with her right index finger to the ulnar styloid on her left hand*):   It's so sore; it hurts terribly. The pain wakes me up in the middle of the night. It's worst in the morning. Sometimes I feel better later in the day, but it takes me a long time to get started.

Last week my doctor reduced my prednisone from 7.5 to 5 mg, and the next day the pain was much worse. I thought the doctor here would be able to help me. But I don't think I'll ever get better; I'm afraid that I'll keep going downhill. I feel depressed and sad all the time.

LIAISON PSYCHIATRIST: Do you work?

MRS. E.: I used to. Six years ago, before this began, I was very active. But now my doctor feels I should take it easy. I couldn't work anyhow.

LIAISON PSYCHIATRIST: Are you able to take care of your family?

MRS. E.: I try, but I'm so tired all the time. I don't want to do anything. I don't even feel like eating. My family doesn't feel the way they used to about me. My husband's so distant; I don't know him any more.

LIAISON PSYCHIATRIST: Are you able to have sex with your husband?

MRS. E.: No, I'm so sick, too sick for sex. I have too much pain.

Mrs. E. then left, and the conference continued.

LIAISON PSYCHIATRIST: I think some of Mrs. E.'s symptoms are suggestive of depression.

DR. V. (*rheumatologist*): Night arousal from pain, fatigue, decreased appetite and libido may all stem from the systemic effects of rheumatoid arthritis. Furthermore, the early morning stiffness and pain she complained of and her feelings of hopelessness about a cure and bleak outlook for the future are often part of the rheumatoid picture.

LIAISON PSYCHIATRIST: But isn't she overreacting? The pain she complained about in her ulnar styloid certainly seemed out of keeping with the appearance of the joint. And isn't it striking that she had increased symptoms the very day after such a slight reduction in her steroid dosage?

DR. V.: No. She wasn't overreacting or being dramatic; she was demonstrating a classic finding in rheumatoid arthritis patients.

LIAISON PSYCHIATRIST: What you're saying is that Mrs. E.'s sadness and tearfulness are appropriate to her advanced illness. Obviously, she's suffered a loss of function, beauty, youth, well-being, and hope of recovery. It's interesting to see the depressive symptom constellation against this patient's array of medical symptoms. But that doesn't alter the fact that this patient is experiencing significant psychological distress. Would you have referred Mrs. E. for psychiatric help after you had elicited details of her life situation?

DR. V.: No. I would offer her a long-term continuing relationship, but I wouldn't attempt to go beyond the psychological issues she raises spontaneously. The illness is chronic, with increasing disability that will eventually leave her crippled, so a relationship of trust is required to prevent such patients from "shopping" for false hopes.

LIAISON PSYCHIATRIST: It seems to me that Mrs. E. has given up much function because she was encouraged by her physician to "take it easy." I think, too, that she felt he would condone her decision to stop having sexual relations with her husband, because she was "so sick."

DR. V.: You interrogated the patient to get that data. I wouldn't have asked her about that. A doctor with a busy medical practice doesn't have time to ask questions like that.

LIAISON PSYCHIATRIST: It's my feeling that Mrs. E. is afraid that she'll hurt herself if she returns to work and sex. I think her marked sex and work inhibitions need further investigation. I'm a little surprised that neither her physician nor the patient herself has inquired about psychiatric help.

Dr. V. left at this point, and the conference continued.

LIAISON PSYCHIATRIST (*to liaison fellows and psychiatric residents*): You've had an opportunity to see and listen to a patient with a specific illness, and a physician whose approach to such patients would be considered typical of specialists in this field. The limitations that were evident in the services Dr. V. provides for his patients underscore the problem we face in trying to foster adequate psychological care for the "normal" medically ill patient.

I think it's interesting that Dr. V. viewed the probing of Mrs. E.'s feelings as an interrogation. But he didn't see anything wrong with exposing her knee joints at a conference in order to demonstrate her range of motion, or with discussing aspects of her medical care in front of her; these things are done all the time. In other words, talking about the patient or exposing part of her body is perfectly acceptable, but asking her about her painful feelings is viewed as an assault on her dignity.

The rheumatologist felt that Mrs. E.'s depressive symptoms were part and parcel of her medical illness, and were not amenable to psychological understanding and treatment. He may have been wrong. The liaison psychiatrist felt that her symptoms, while they may have been in part a reaction to her medical illness, should nevertheless have been understood and dealt with from a psychological point of view as well. He may have been wrong. Some of these symptoms may be inherent in systemic rheumatoid arthritis; on the other hand, they may be universal psychological reactions to the arthritic process. One point emerges clearly: further investigation of the physical and psychological aspects of Mrs. E.'s illness —and their interrelationship—is essential. This teaching conference underscored the dangers of premature closure in considering a patient's symptoms.

Residents and liaison fellows were taught the basic principles and central clinical issues of liaison psychiatry, did two or three consultations per week, and attended weekly liaison conferences and ombudsman rounds. They were also encouraged to run a nurses' conference, to treat psychologically disturbed medically ill patients in their clinic practice, and to participate in clinical research projects.

The Department of Psychiatry was able to arrange for psychiatric nurses from the inpatient service to assist in the management of disturbed patients on the medical and surgical wards. Moreover, we were given permission to move patients, when possible, to a holding area on the psychiatric inpatient service where they could be provided with close medical supervision until their psychiatric crisis was over. The Department of Medicine and Psychiatry also drew up plans for a room with two beds on the medical service that would be available for the management of disturbed patients directly on the medical ward and that would be staffed jointly by Psychiatry and Medicine.

Liaison attendings, who were reimbursed for their services by third-party payers, were hired to care for medical patients in the ambulatory renal dialysis and transplant units. In short, we were able to buy psychiatric care for a group of patients who lived outside the district served by the Department of Psychiatry, and who had not been referred, without inflicting an increased patient load on psychiatric residents.

Since the psychiatrist should be able to treat the psychological problems of the medically ill, talk with medical doctors, be conversant with organic brain syndromes, and be competent in the use of psychotropic drugs for the medically ill, the Department of Psychiatry agreed to provide a core curriculum for medical students and psychiatric residents that would be heavily invested with liaison issues. The well-trained psychiatrist has a broader base than simply the psychotherapy of the neurotic.

Comment.   If liaison psychiatry is to accomplish its task, it must build an alliance with its own Department of Psychiatry. Moreover, liaison psychiatry must bring the Department of Psychiatry face to face with the hospital in which it lives and works. The liaison psychiatrist tactfully attempts to move the ship of state to a more central location, and to encourage his psychiatric colleagues to consider liaison issues in their own operations. Without this alliance he has no mandate; he is a man without a professional identity.

THE HOSPITAL ADMINISTRATION

Regardless of whether the hospital moves to an industrial bureaucracy or remains an advisory bureaucracy, only the hospital administration can ensure adequate psychological care for its patients. Unless the liaison psychiatrist is given the authority and trappings to disseminate the knowledge and experience necessary to affect patient care, unless he is recognized within the hospital hierarchy as an ambassador with portfolio, he will remain a doctor-chaser, an ear-clutcher, a patient-chaser pleading to be heard. It is our feeling that the industrial bureaucracy offers the liaison psychiatrist the only setting in which he can be assured of an opportunity to work independently of the personal predilections of individuals. It seems obvious, therefore, that rather than try to shape one tooth of the "comb" at a time, he must make a central thrust to influence the apex of the "tree."

What keeps the liaison psychiatrist going in the face of overwhelming odds is his deep conviction that the application of psychological principles would have a meaningful impact on every aspect of the patient's care—the course and, at times, the outcome of his illness, his convalescence, the morale and orientation of his caretakers, and the very climate and spirit of the hospital. The liaison psychiatrist must imbue the administration with that conviction.

For, whatever form it takes, only the administration can make it possible for the liaison psychiatrist to cut across departmental lines to see to it that training programs are enriched with sufficient psychological knowledge to ensure each patient the quantity and quality of psychological care he is entitled to.

Some progress has been made toward that end. As mentioned earlier, the administration has long required every drug overdose patient to have a psychiatric assessment before leaving the intensive care unit and, more recently, made psychiatric clearance mandatory for all candidates for "life island" therapy. The next logical step would be to make psychiatric clearance mandatory for other high-risk patients, for example, candidates for open heart surgery (where the mortality rate is known to be higher among depressed patients); patients who present diagnostic problems, and where some doubt exists about the need for surgery; and patients who have repeated hospital admissions, apparently as a consequence of self-abuse through neglect. Psychiatric clearance in such cases should not depend on the whim of a patient, a physician, or a department. Rather, psychological assessment of these patient groups—and others yet to be identified—should be regarded as an intrinsic part of patient evaluation and management in the contemporary teaching hospital. This may come to pass when the hospital administration officially recognizes that improved psychological care of the medically ill diminishes the frequency and length of hospitalization, and postpones chronicity.

Epilogue

Reading this fine book is a sobering experience for those who care *about* patients as well as for them. Drs. Strain and Grossman have made it impossible for us to avoid seeing that, even in the felicitous and supportive environment of Montefiore Hospital and Medical Center, there is little more than lip service paid to a given of modern medical care whose premise is that, because the psyche and the soma are so intertwined, we must minister to both, and that their separation in the care of the patient is damaging to that care.

The usefulness of this primer lies in the fact that the authors have delineated the obstacles to the introduction of psychological care in the traditional hospital setting and have proposed specific steps and mechanisms by which the organization of in-hospital care can be restructured to accommodate holistic medicine. The study of this primer by every doctor who cares for patients and by every professional who purports to be concerned with the delivery of good care is the minimum initial step that needs to be taken.

I must note, however, that if we are to have more than the "islands of excellence" to which the authors have referred and extend their characteristics to care of all people, we are going to have to tackle matters underlying medical education and health care delivery that are only hinted at in this book. Because if everyone agrees that proper care of patients requires that we deal with both psychological and physiological needs and the knowledge and the teaching techniques are available, we must ask why it is so difficult to accomplish this goal. We must question why—even at Montefiore, where work with intractable chronic diseases taught us the importance of the emotional and psychological components of illness, where programs such as Home Care and After Care are testimonials to this knowledge and experience, and where administrative policy has prepared the institution to welcome liaison psychiatry—the necessary integration of disciplines has not been more widely achieved.

The answers lie in the characteristics of the medical system in this country—the selection of health professionals, their career goals and objectives, their educational environment, and the way in which medical care is organized and financed. Examination of any of these considerations explains why liaison psychiatry is enmeshed in a struggle and why the road it travels will continue to be a very difficult one. The goals and objectives of both house officers and their teachers in undergraduate as well as post-graduate medical education, and the rewards they seek, just do not lie in such activities as improving care through consideration of the psychological factors of illness. By rewards, I mean status, recognition, money, and successful practice. In view of the rat race that characterizes academe, harassed house officers have a desperate need to establish priorities. The amount of time and energy necessary to undertake this additional major facet of patient care just cannot compete with more clearly recognized and establishment-approved professional activities such as concern for the practice of good scientific medicine, attention to proper laboratory procedures, employment of definitive surgery, use of appropriate drugs, and so forth.

The authors comment on the receptivity of nurses and social workers to the liaison psychiatry program and relate how eager they are to lend their considerable skills to its implementation. Quite clearly, the program enhances their operations and meets some of the self-serving goals of nursing and social work—factors that must be favorable if any professional is to devote time and energy, always in short supply, to additional activities.

For the psychiatrist, this is the area of his life's work. Indeed, it is what he gets paid to do, and the value to him as well as to the patient is quite clear. Yet, liaison psychiatry is sufficiently apart from the mainstream of many academic psychiatric programs that it has had some fair amount of difficulty finding its place within psychiatry—almost comparable to the difficulty it has had being accepted by medicine, surgery, and other specialties. While this crossing of lines may be good for patient care, nice, clear, sharp career lines, goals, and accomplishments are delicious for professionals and despite the rhetoric, they find multidisciplined situations uncomfortable and anxiety-producing.

One of the critical handicaps to holistic medicine dealt with time and again in this volume is the fact that doctors are just as human as their patients, have the same range of psychological difficulties as their patients, do and need to protect their vulnerability and to deny their inadequacies as do their patients. One consideration that stands in the way of the doctor really involving himself with his patients and dealing with his patients' fears, anxieties, and feelings has been that there is a heavy price to be paid by the health professional who gets to know his patient in the way you must know him to be able to support him psychologically. This kind of involvement is very costly to the physician not only in terms of his time, but also as far as his own psychic energy is concerned. Only a physician who has carried patients and families through calamitous illness knows the pain and stress that this support can produce for him, personally. The immense technology of scientific medicine, the endless tests and procedures, are used by the doctor not only to examine the patient's pathology, but also as a barrier between him and the patient for whom he can "care" without becoming painfully involved. While it is true that the physician and the surgeon must maintain a sufficient distance from the patient so that their objectivity is not impaired, the distances are often greater than necessary because that is more comfortable for the doctor, even if it is less useful for the patient.

Further, if one examines the way medical care is paid for, it is obvious that insufficient thought has been given to the need to treat psychological problems along with physical illness. It is interesting to note that it has been possible to bring about an effective program of psychological support where there were specific financial provisions for people suffering from renal disease.* However, the whole present system of reimbursement represents a serious block to the treatment of psychological problems, because physical illness and its manifestations are universally recognized as needing care and, therefore, money, but emotional illness as part of physical illness and its threats to a patient are only peripherally recognized.

The comments about some of the underlying reasons why medicine in a teaching hospital often couples spectacular lifesaving capabilities with minimal regard for psychological considerations should, if anything, make this book more important for all who care about or are involved with patient care and education of health professionals. The introduction of psychological support for hospitalized patients should not require the presence of a unique Chairman of Medicine who, almost against the traditions of his training, is sensitive and dedicated enough to commit his time, energy, and prestige as an ombudsman and who, once having started on this path, inexorably moved to the development of "islands of excellence" in medicine. Progress toward holistic medicine cannot rest on so slender a reed as the humanism of individual physicians. The ideal will never even be approached unless it is fostered by administrative bias and buttressed by administrative policy and budget lines. For the well-being of our patients, we now assure standards of hygiene within the hospital through the services of an infectious disease staff, which has the cooperation of all personnel and departments. It should be possible to assure minimal standards of mental hygiene in much the same way.

The millenium has not come, and easy solutions are not at hand. The fact that we cannot quickly reshape medical education, the health care delivery system, and the methods of reimbursement does not relieve those of us who have stewardship for patients of our responsibilities—it merely

---

* Under Public Law 92-603, Medicare payments of up to $500 per year are available for psychiatric services to all chronic renal dialysis patients and to all renal transplant patients for one year postsurgery regardless of age.

makes the challenge more difficult. It seems to me that Drs. Strain and Grossman have given us a clear presentation of how things are now, as well as an outline of the ways in which we can help doctors, nurses, social workers, and other health professionals express what is within most of us—that is the wanting and the need to do good. We must move rapidly to incorporate what is in this text into the texture of medical care and medical education. For, no matter how brilliant our science and technology, if that is all we apply, we do only half the job.

Martin Cherkasky

Index

Abdominal neoplasms, and depression, 73
Acute agitation, recommended drugs for, 113–114
"Acute situational" reactions, 9
Adaptation
  to deficits in mental functioning, 41
  to illness and hospitalization, 33–35
  to psychological stress, 29
"Affective neutrality," 5
Alcohol, 39
Alexander, F., 4, 10, 54–55, 56–57, 58–59, 62, 152
Ambivalence, 31, 82
Ambulatory medical services, See Liaison program, at Montefiore Hospital
Amputation, 26, 122
Anger, as maladaptive reaction of psychiatrist, 46–47
Angina
  and personality traits, 153
  and REM sleep, 61
Animal models, 60–154
Anxiety
  in coronary patients, 159
  in postoperative patients, 133
  preoperative, 123–125, 130–131
  recommended drugs for, 114

Anxiety (cont.)
  role of fantasy in, See Fear
Asthma, 55
Attitudes of physician, unconscious
  as destructive force, 142–144
  as "indestructible," 141–142
  as "powerful healer," 139–141, 147
  and response to dying patient, 138–147
Autonomic nervous system, See Alexander, F.; Coronary heart disease, initiating mechanisms in and predisposing factors in
Autonomy, loss of, 26

Balint, M., 8, 10, 106
Beecher, H. K., 94, 98–99, 105, 106
Bereavement, 154
Bibring, G., 8, 10, 23, 24, 36
Biochemical factors, as genesis of disease, 61, 65
Biofeedback experiments, 60
Bisexual conflict, 26, 164
Body image
  and infantile experience, 21
  and pain, 25
  preoccupation with, 81
  and surgery, 127

Body language
in lieu of verbalization, 35
Brain syndromes
acute, 40
chronic, 40
denial of, 38
evaluation, 42
treatment, 47
Bureaucracy, in hospital, 171–172, 184

Cannon, W., 54
Caplan, G., 8, 10
Cardiac surgery, impact of preoperative anxiety and depression on outcome of, 130–131
Cardiovascular disease
and affects, 155
and personality, 152
use of psychotropic drugs with, 118
and stress, 155
Castration anxiety, 26–27
in coronary patients, 167
management of, 160–167
in surgical patients, 124
"Catastrophic" reaction, 41
Central nervous system diseases, *See* Brain syndromes
use of psychotropic drugs with, 120–121
Character reactions
in coronary patients, 159
maladaptive, 34
Classification of psychotropic drugs, 109–110
Clinical competence, 5–7
Cognition, evaluation of, 44
Colitis, 58
Communication
breakdown in surgical service, 125
of psychiatric assessment, 21–22
Conflict, *See* Stresses
Conversion reaction, 65
and hypochondriasis, 80
and pain, 98

Coronary heart disease
convalescent problems in, 162–167
initiating mechanisms in, 154–157
predisposing factors in, 152–154
and psychological reactions, 158–162
and sexual functioning, 155–156
and work inhibitions, 157
Coronary personality
biological basis, 152
characteristics, 152
psychological testing, 153
Critchley, M., 94, 105
Crohn's disease, 58
Crying, 26
Cushing's syndrome, and depression 72

Decompensation, 42
Defensive reaction, in psychological stress, 28
Defense measures, used by medical staff, 144–145
Delirium, 40
in postoperative patients, 133
Delirium tremens, 39
Dementia, 40
Denial, 124; *See also* Ego defenses
Depression
and abdominal neoplasms, 73
in coronary patients, 159
drug-induced, 73–74
and endocrinopathies, 73–74
evaluating, in the medical patient, 64–75
"masked," 77–78
neurotic characterological, 71–72
in postoperative patients, 134
treatment of, 71–72, 114–115
Depressive illness, 74
diagnosis of, 66–67
psychological symptoms of, 64–65
somatic symptoms of, 65, 80

Depressive illness (*cont.*)
treatment of, 67–68
Deutsch, F., 54, 62
Diagnosis, formulation, 23
Diagnostic and Statistical Manual of
Mental Disorders, 91
Diagnostic tools, in organic brain
syndromes, 42–45
Displacement, 82
Distractability, 43, 146
Dreams, 61
Drug-drug effect, 115–116
Drug-induced depressions, 73–74
Drugs, psychotropic
classification of, 109–110
effects on elderly patient, 117–118
overdosage of, 117
overuse and underuse of, 110–111
side effects, 116–117, 118
solubility of, 117
therapeutic potency of, 11–13
use of, with physiological disorders,
118–121
Drug withdrawal, 117
Dying patient, physician's response to,
138–145

Ego alien symptoms, 41
Ego controls, 43
Ego defenses
in acute and chronic illness, 30
reactions to undermining of, 14
Ego functions, assessment of, 42–43
Ego psychology, in assessment of
organic brain syndrome,
41–43
Ego regression, 43
Elderly patient
effect of drugs on, 117–118
and organic brain syndromes, 38,
40
and separation anxiety, 26
Endocrinopathies, and depression,
72–73
Engel, G. L., 8, 10, 40, 50, 58, 62,
97, 106

Environmental intervention, in coro-
nary patients, 162
Epilepsy, 43
Exhibitionism, 21, 200

Family, response to illness, 16, 20,
67, 154
Fantasy
castration, 26, 124, 167
control of, 35
denial of reality in, 33
hypochondriasis, 83
object loss, 26
passive feminine, 26, 164
sexual, 26
unconscious, 35, 139
Father image, 29
Fear
of loss of control of bodily functions, 26
of loss of love and approval, 26
of loss of love object, 30, 144; *See
also* Separation anxiety
of loss or injury to body parts,
26–27; *See also* Castration
anxiety
of pain, 27
of strangers, 25
of surgery, 26, 124
of terminal illness, 138
Freud, S., 4, 41, 50
Friedman, M., 59, 62, 152, 154, 169
Frustration
of internist, 139
in pain, 98
of psychiatrist, 146
in terminal illness, 138

Gain, secondary, 72, 81, 98
Gastrointestinal
Alexander's formulation, 55
gastric secretion, 56
in hypochrondriasis, 78
mucous colitis, 58
psychological influence on, 61

Gastrointestinal (*cont.*)
  ulcerative colitis, 58
Genitals, 27, 167
Geriatrics, 26, 117
Graves disease, 56, 57
Grief reactions, 68–71
  distinguished from depressive illness, 68, 70
  as response to real object loss, 154
Guilt
  in fear of retaliation, 27
  in hypochondriasis, 83
  in pain, 96

Hackett, T. P., 130, 136, 148, 155, 169
Hallucinations
  as ego function, 43
  olfactory, 46
  organic mental syndrome, 43
Helplessness, 125, 144
Hellerstein, H. K., 155, 156, 169
Hepatic disease
  cholestatic jaundice, 117, 119
  complications
    with antidepressants, 119
    with morphine, 119
    with paraldehyde, 119
    with phenothiazines, 119
  use of psychotropic drugs with, 119
Henry, J. P., 61, 62–63, 154, 169
Hinkle, L. E., 152, 169
Hofer, M. A., 60–61, 62, 154, 169
Hollingshead, A. B., 79, 91, 98, 106
Home, as object loss, 26
Homosexuality, 26
Hormones
  in depression, 67
  in psychomatic research, 60
Hospitalization
  psychological stress of, 24–27
  successful adaption to, 33–34
Humor, 124
Hyperparathyroidism, and depression, 72

Hypertension, 57–58
  and drug-induced depression, 74
  and personality traits, 152
Hyperthyroidism, 57
Hypochondriasis, 76, 82–83
  classification of, 77–78
  and depression, 77–78
  diagnosis and clinical description of, 78–80
  diagnostic types, 83–87
  differential diagnosis of, 80–82
  as transitional state, 82–83
  treatment of, 87–91
Hypothyroidism, and depression, 72
Hysteria, conversion, 80, 98

Illness, physical
  and attitudes of psychiatrist, 5–6, 7
  psychological factors in, 4, 54–56
  psychological reactions to, 7, 12
  somato-psychic effects of, 39, 51–52, 55–56
  and stress, 59
  and unresolved neurotic conflict, 54–55, 57–58
Illness and hospitalization
  patients' response to, 56
  psychological stress of, 24–27
  successful adaptation to, 33–34
Impotence, 156
Insomnia, recommended drugs for, 114
Interview
  of patient, 18–19
  scope of, in psychiatric assessment, 12–13

Joint pain, *See* rheumatoid arthritis
Judgment
  organic mental syndrome, 143
  for surgery, 135

Kahana, R., 8, 10, 23, 36

Kidney disease, *See* renal disease
Kimball, C. P., 130, 136
Klein, D. F., 66, 67, 74, 75
Klerman, G., 74
Korsakoff's psychosis, 45
Krystal, H., 24, 36
Kübler-Ross, E., 147, 148

"La belle indifference," 80, 98
Leukemia, 14, 142
Levopromazine, 104
Liaison model, of coronary heart
     disease, 151–170
Liaison modular unit, 195
Liaison program, at Montefiore Hospital
     in ambulatory medical care, 194–
         196
     in Department of Medicine, 188–
         194
     in Department of Psychiatry,
         203–208
     in Nursing Department, 198–203
     and renal dialysis and transplant
         patients, 195–196
     in Social Service Department,
         196–197
Liaison psychiatry, 1, 3–10
     and alliance with other departments, 185–208
     goals of, 9
     and hospital administration, 208–
         209
Libido, 65
Librium, 110
Lipowski, Z. J., 147, 148
Lipsitt, D., 77, 83, 90, 91
Lithium, 68
Looking, *See* voyeurism
Loss
     of autonomy, 25
     of love, 26
     of self-esteem in hospitalized patient, 28–29

Magical thinking, 129

Malingering, 81, 99
Manic-depressive disorder (bi-polar
     depression), 68
Martin Luther King, Jr., Health Center, 195
Masculinity, concerns about, 164
Masochism
     in hypochondriasis, 83
     in pain, 96
Masturbation
     as defense, 124
     as exhibitionism, 17
Mattis Dementia Rating Scale, 45
Medical depressions, 67, 72–73
Medicine, future of, 211–214
Memory
     Korsakoff's psychosis, 45
     measures of, 45
     in organic mental syndrome, 43
Mendelson, M., 13, 22
Mental functioning
     assessment of, 19, 42–47
     coping with deficits in, 41
     deficits in, and stress, 41
     psychoanalytic model of, 42–43
Mental Status Examination, 42, 44–
         46
Meperidine, 101
Metabolism and drug response, 104,
         115
Miller, N., 60, 62
Mirsky, A., 56, 62
Montefiore Hospital and Medical
         Center
     admission rate, 172
     coronary care unit, 155, 157, 163
     liaison program, 188–200, 202–
         204, 207
     medical clinic study, 79, 130
     neurology service in, 178
     oncology service in, 178
     patient advocates at, 181–183
     patient population, 175–176
     percentage of private patients in,
         175
     psychiatric service in, 182–183
     surgical service in, 177

Montefiore Hospital and Medical Center (*cont.*)
  training program, 178–180
  turnover of nurses in, 180
Mood
  affect on cardiac function, 155
  drugs, 114
Morphine, 110
Motor control, 43
Mourning, 49, 154
Multiple sclerosis, 18

Narcissistic integrity, threats to, 25, 31; *See also* Omnipotence
Neuodermatitis, 59
Neurotic characterological depressions, 67, 71–72
Norton, J., 82, 92, 148
Noyes, A. P., 106
Nursing-liaison teaching conference, 200–202
Nursing personnel, 180, 183
  liaison program for, 198–203

Object
  disillusionment with, 25
  identification with, 162
  loss of, 25–26
Object relations, 29–30, 33; *See also* Ego functions, assessment of; Regression in, 29; Relationship, doctor-patient
Obsessional neurosis, 81
Omnipotence of physician, unresolved feelings of in patients and physicians, 101, 139–144, 147
Organic mental syndromes, 37–39
  classification of, 40
  clinical features of, 39–42
  diagnosis of, 42–47
  treatment of, 47–50
Outpatient Department, *See* Liaison program, at Montefiore Hospital

Pain
  congenital absence of, 94, 95
  as conversion reaction, 98
  genetic factors in, 95–96
  and perception, 96
  in postoperative patient, 133–134
  psychobiological aspects of, 93–95
  as psychological stress, 96–97
  psychopathological reactions to, 97
  and stimulus, 94
  and threshold, 94–96
  and tolerance, 95, 97
  undiagnosed, 98
Pain management, 100–103
  guidelines for, 103–105
  in terminal illness, 101, 105
  underuse of analgesics in, 101–102
"Pain-prone" patient, 97
Passivity, 164
Patient advocates, 181–182
Patient care, 3, 6–8
  and holistic approach, 3–5, 188
  and rotation of staff, 7, 173–175
Patient evaluation, on surgical service, 126–131
Penis, 17
Peptic ulcer, 55, 56, 57, 59, 61
  and personality traits, 152
Perception, 43
Personality traits
  and coronary disease, 59, 152–153
  and hypertension, 152
  and illness, 54, 57
  and maladaptation, 27–28, 159
  and peptic ulcer, 152
Perversion, 96
Pessimism, 64
Phobia, *See* Coronary heart disease, and sexual functioning; and work inhibitions
Placebo, 98
Pleasure from pain, 96
Prange, A. G., Jr., 112, 121
Premenstrual tension, 72

Preparation for surgery, 131
Prevention schemes, 9
Professional training, and clinical competence, 6–7
Projection, 144–145
Psychiatric assessment, in medical setting
clinical example of, 19–21
communication of, *See* Communication
contrasted with traditional setting, 11
and patient chart, 15–16
scope of interview in, 12, 13
and ward culture, 17–18
Psychiatric consultation, requests for evaluating, 13
in the medical service, 177–178
in the surgical service, 177
Psychiatric interview, expanded
and evaluating the doctor, 13–15
and evaluating the family, 17
and evaluating the nurse, 16–17
Psychiatrist, liaison
contrasted with consulting, 9, 185
and dying patient, 145–147
functions of, in surgical service, 134–136
maladaptive reactions in, 146–147
role of, 8–9, 71, 168
and structural change, 185–187
and teaching conferences, 187–188
Psychoanalytic model of mental functioning, 42–43
Psychogenic pain, 94, 97–100
and depression, 98
Psychological care, 7–8
and model of prevention, 9
team approach to, 8–9, 182–184
Psychological dysfunction
in coronary patients, 157–167
organic precipitants of, 37–50
Psychological intervention
in coronary patients, 160–167
and pharmacological treatment, 108–122

Psychological intervention (*cont.*)
in surgical patients, 131–134
Psychological reactions
to coronary disease, 160–167
to illness and hospitalization, 23–36
to pain, 96–97
to stress, 28–30
Psychology, of the medically ill
clinical correlations of, 33–35
theories in, 23–27
Psychopharmacological intervention
in coronary patients, 161
Psychopharmacological treatment, 108–122
Psychophysiological reactions, 59–61, 80–81
Psychosomatic medicine, 54–59
new areas of research in, 59–61
Psychosomatic Specificity, 55
Punishment, pain as choice of, 96

Regression
in hospitalized patient, 27, 29–30
innate property, 29
and organic brain syndromes, 41
"in service of recovery," 33
Reiser, M., 56, 62, 153, 155, 169
Relationship, doctor-patient, 5, 31–33, 99, 132
and rotation, 172–175
Renal disease
ambulatory care, 195
use of psychotropic drugs, 120
Resistance to teaching, 188
Response of physician
to dying patient, 138–148
to intervention by psychiatrist, 145–146
Rheumatoid arthritis, 58, 59, 204–207
Risk factors, in coronary heart disease, 152
Role models, 2, 179
Romano, J., 8, 10

Rosenman, R. H., 59, 62, 152, 154, 169
Rotation
of hospital staff, 173–175
of patients, 173

Sachar, E. J., 75, 101, 106
Sadism, 142
St. Bernard, 4
Saunders, C., 105, 107
Schildkraut, J., 71, 75
Schizophrenia, 81
Sedatives, 114
Seductiveness, 192
Self esteem, 28
Self sacrifice, 82
Separation anxiety, 25–26
in surgical patients, 124
Sexual functioning, and coronary heart disease, 155–156
Shader, R. I., 121
Shame, 27
Shands, 46, 50
Shapiro, A. K., 106
Shock treatment, 67
Sleep, 61
disturbances of, 65
Social workers, role of, 180–182, 183
Somatization, 83
Stelazine, 9
Stress
and childhood experiences, 29
clinical variations of, 27–28
hormones sensitive to, 60
of illness and hospitalization, 24–27
and neuroendocrine system, 60
on physician, 31–33, 138
on psychiatrist, 145–146
psychological reactions to, 28–30
and somatic disease, 59, 60
on surgical patient, 123–125
and "temporary" hypochondriacs, 81–82
Suicide, 70

Superego disturbance, 27, 43
Supportive approach, in hypochondriasis, 87–90
Surgical patient
and postoperative psychological problems, 133–134
preoperative psychological preparation of, 131–133
stresses on, 123–125
Symbolic equation, 167
Szasz, T. S., 94, 105

Tact, 208
Talland, G. A., 50
Teaching conference, 187–188
in Department of Medicine, 190–194
in Department of Nursing, 200–202
and Department of Psychiatry, 204–207
in Outpatient Department, 195
Teaching hospital
defects in organization and operation of, 7, 171–172
and nursing care, 180
and social service staff, 180–181
Team approach
in psychiatric ward, 182–184
to psychological care, 8–9
responsibility for, 150
Terminal illness
and hypochondriasis, 82
management of pain in, 101, 105
and organic brain syndrome, 40
Thaler, M., 56, 62
Thorazine (Chlorpromazine), 109
Transference, counter transference, 31
Treatment
of anxiety, *See* Anxiety; Castration anxiety, management of
of depression, 67–68, 71–72, 114–115
of hypochondriasis, 90–91

Treatment (*cont.*)
  of organic brain syndromes, 47
  psychopharmacological, 108–122

Ulcerative colitis, 55, 58, 59
Ulcer, peptic, 55–56

Valium, 110, 114, 118
Verbalization role of, 16
Viral illness, and depression, 73
Voyeurism, 200

Wallerstein, R. S., 56, 62
Wechsler Adult Intelligence Scale
  Similarities Subtest, 45
Weight loss, 65
Weiner, H., 56, 57, 60–61, 62, 153,
  154, 169
Weisman, A. D., 148
Weiss, J. M., 61, 63
Withdrawal, abandonment of patient
  by transfer, 144
Work inhibitions, and coronary heart
  disease, 157

Zohman, L., 157, 170